The Dentist's Guide to Atraumatic Extractions

One book, one tree: In support of reforestation worldwide and to address the climate crisis, for every book sold Quintessence Publishing will plant a tree (https://onetreeplanted.org/).

Library of Congress Cataloging-in-Publication Data

Names: Mason, William E. (Periodontist), author.
Title: The dentist's guide to atraumatic extractions / William E. Mason.
Description: Batavia, IL : Quintessence Publishing, [2023] | Includes bibliographical references and index. | Summary: "This book explains the atraumatic extraction technique and demonstrates this technique step by step for every tooth in the mouth"-- Provided by publisher.
Identifiers: LCCN 2022039386 | ISBN 9781647241391 (paperback)
Subjects: MESH: Tooth Extraction--methods
Classification: LCC RK531 | NLM WU 605 | DDC 617.6/6--dc23/eng/20221109
LC record available at https://lccn.loc.gov/2022039386

A CIP record for this book is available from the British Library.
ISBN: 9781647241391

QUINTESSENCE PUBLISHING USA

Quintessence Publishing Co, Inc
411 N Raddant Road
Batavia, IL 60510
www.quintpub.com

5 4 3 2 1

Editor: Leah Huffman
Design & production: Sue Zubek

Printed in Croatia

The Dentist's Guide to Atraumatic Extractions

WILLIAM E. MASON, DDS, MS

Adjunct Clinical Assistant Professor of Dentistry
University of Michigan School of Dentistry
Ann Arbor, Michigan

Private Practice
Saginaw, Michigan

QUINTESSENCE PUBLISHING

Berlin | Chicago | Tokyo
Barcelona | London | Milan | Mexico City | Paris | Prague | Seoul | Warsaw
Beijing | Istanbul | Sao Paulo | Zagreb

Contents

Preface

This book is for general practitioners, periodontists, oral surgeons, endodontists, pediatric dentists, and prosthodontists interested in improving their extraction technique and their ability to preserve bone following extraction. It is the culmination of having placed more than 5,000 implants, mostly one at a time. Many of these procedures involved a prior extraction.

In the early 1990s, when dental implants were becoming recognized as a viable option for tooth replacement, most patients presented with the tooth removed already. The result was a large ridge defect that required guided bone regeneration (GBR) before implant placement. I asked myself: Are we extracting teeth or bone? Because the bone was being removed in order to facilitate tooth removal. It just didn't make sense to me that for the sake of extracting teeth as quickly as possible, bone was being sacrificed.

I thought, why not remove tooth structure—which will be removed anyway—to make space for tooth removal, instead of removing bone to make space for tooth removal? I am not extracting bone, am I? Because bone is difficult to replace.

My hope and goal is to pass on these techniques to the dental profession to reduce our patients' postoperative discomfort, to maintain the residual ridges, and to help improve final outcomes. Enjoy!

Acknowledgments

I would like to thank my parents—William G. Mason, MD, and Suzanne T. Mason—for creating a loving family environment and instilling a work ethic with expectations. Also, my mentors Billy Smith, DDS, MS, and Frank Rugani, DDS, were instrumental in my early years of practice. They embodied professionalism and excellence in dentistry and served as models for me. My grandfather, William J.B. Mason, DDS, provided my first exposure to dentistry, which proved to be both a positive and lasting one.

I would like to thank my wonderful wife, Ann, for her patience and support. She not only gives me space to pursue my projects and passions but also offers feedback and encouragement along the way.

I am fortunate to be a member of the Dean's Faculty at the University of Michigan School of Dentistry, teaching monthly in the Graduate Periodontics Clinic. I want to thank Dr Hom-Lay Wang, Dr Will Giannobile, and Dr Laurie McCauley for inviting me to contribute to the education of the residents. I am truly honored to have that privilege and to be continually inspired by all of the leaders at the school, as well as the residents.

I would like to thank my daughters—Dr Chelsea Mason, a general dentist, and Dr Suzanne Mason-Dennis, a periodontist—for motivating me to keep abreast of the latest developments in dentistry. They are inspirational and represent the exceptional young practitioners in our profession.

Also, this book would have been much more difficult to complete without my photography assistant, Sophie McConnell. She stepped up when needed—always with a smile on her face. In addition, Kristina Fanning was my go-to person for organizing and transmitting the transcript and photographs. I truly appreciate her technical skills and patience.

I would like to thank my referring doctors and their patients for allowing me to participate in their care. Without them, these ideas would not have come to be.

Finally, the amazing and wonderful staff at Quintessence Publishing—Bryn Grisham, Director of Book Publications, and Leah Huffman, Editorial & Marketing Director—were kind enough to show interest in this topic, accept my manuscript and photographs, and bring it to fruition. I am truly grateful for this opportunity to share these ideas.

Thank you all.

Introduction

My Story

"Frank, *I'm not interested in doing implants; I'm a periodontist! That's for the oral surgeons."* It was 1989, and I had been a practicing periodontist for 5 years. Dr Frank Rugani was a referring dentist who was involved in restoring dental implants. I was not interested in placing dental implants. Dental implants were not included in any periodontal residency at the time, and I had not been trained to place them—only oral surgeons were placing them at that time. But Dr Rugani was very persuasive. He needed a surgical colleague to work with, and I was coerced into spending 3 days at Northwestern Dental School in Chicago at my first Brånemark dental implant training.

Flash forward to 2022, and dental implants make up about 70% of my practice. I have placed over 5,000 dental implants, and the majority of these cases were single tooth extractions with implant placement. Tooth removal has become a big part of my clinical practice.

In the 1990s—the early days of dental implants—my referring dentists would refer patients to me with the tooth or teeth already removed and the ridge already resorbed. For partially edentulous patients or cases with single-tooth replacement, I would have to augment the resorbed ridge, wait 6 months, place the implant, wait another 4 to 6 months, and then uncover and refer the patient back for restoration. Of course as a periodontist I was trained to *save* teeth, not extract them, but as I began to place dental implants, I had to learn how to remove nonrestorable, broken-down teeth—tough extractions for me. I was humbled many, many times, and still am. Over the last 30 years, however, I have developed ways to remove teeth carefully, without raising flaps. Preservation of the bone and its architecture is my priority, along with a gentle technique.

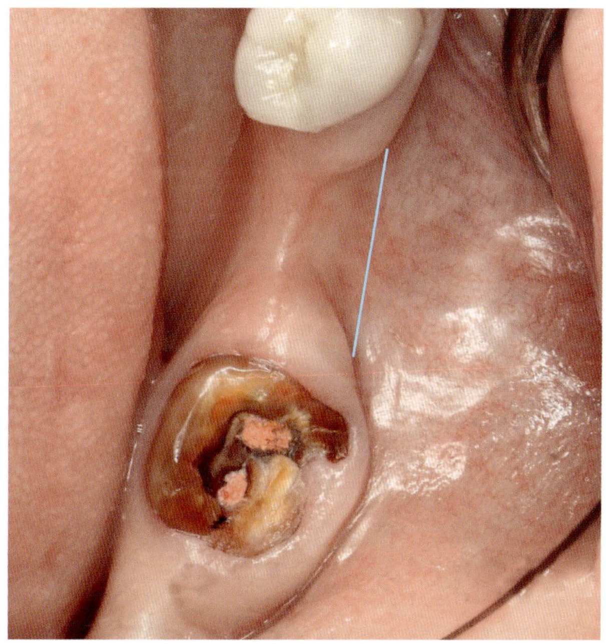

FIG 1-1 Resultant severe vertical and horizontal ridge resorption after extraction of tooth #30, with bone removal to access the roots and without socket preservation. The *blue line* represents the location of the alveolar ridge when tooth #30 was present.

Figure 1-1 shows what I am trying to prevent. But this is what happens when you extract teeth the way you're taught in dental school—with the elevation of full-thickness flap, bone relief, expansion of the sockets, and the use of elevators and forceps. This always results in ridge resorption laterally and vertically; this ridge shrinkage occurs within the first 3 months of healing and is most evident on the buccal.

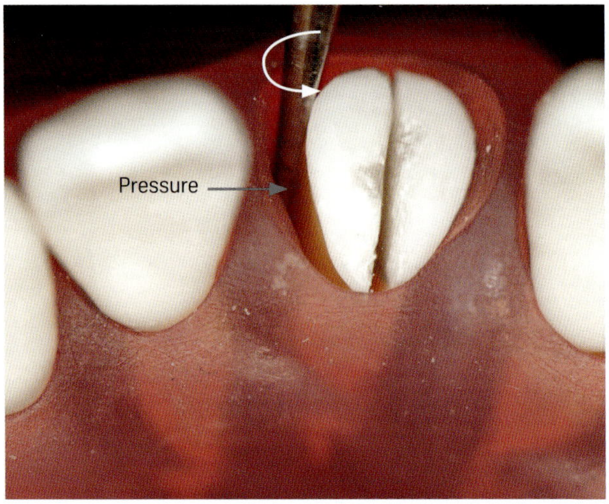

FIG 1-2 Thin elevator inserted into the sulcus and used with a gentle twisting motion to pressure the sectioned root into the created space.

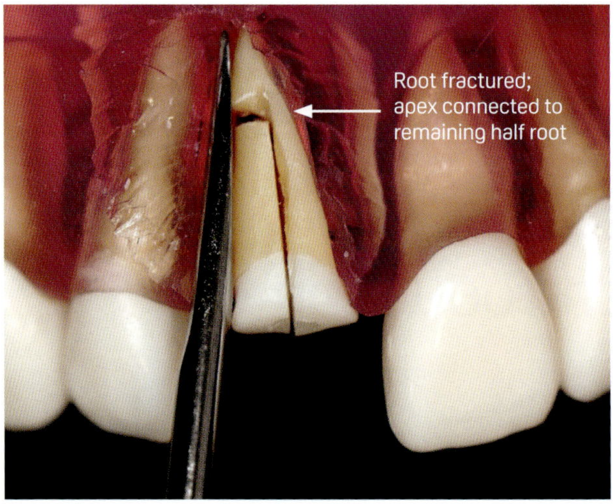

FIG 1-3 Sectioned root fractured during removal because sectioning did not extend all the way to the apex.

And that is why socket preservation is so important. Tooth extraction without socket preservation can lead to food impaction under a fixed restoration, inadequate ridge width for dental implants, thicker flanges on partial or complete dentures, and potential loss of facial support. Atraumatic extraction with socket preservation prevents all this and protects the jaw's original anatomy.

I have noticed that a great deal of research and literature is focused on socket preservation *after* extraction. But the extraction procedure itself has just as much to do with the potential of the socket to be preserved and to heal.[1–5] Many articles and lectures begin their discussion with an empty socket. But what about the trauma caused by the extraction? How long was the extraction procedure? The degree of trauma during the extraction directly affects the postextraction healing.[1,2,4–6]

I am concerned with preservation of the buccal plate. If the buccal plate is damaged, collapse of the socket will occur, mostly from the buccal. Resorption of the buccal plate reduces the arch width and circumference, which can compromise future implant placement because it affects implant positioning and often results in the need for a restorative cantilever.

Dental extractions aren't easy. In fact, they are one of the most difficult and humbling procedures in dentistry. Some of this difficulty is undoubtedly due to the unpredictability of the procedure. Teeth with existing resorption are often ankylosed. Because it is difficult to diagnose ankylosed roots, I always assume that any tooth with resorption is at least partially ankylosed.

Most oral surgery textbooks recommend extraction via large full-thickness buccal and possibly lingual flaps with bone relief.[1,2] Sometimes mesial, distal, and lingual bone relief are also recommended to gain access to the root, followed by luxation and elevation to remove it. These techniques remove teeth fairly quickly, but the long-term effects on ridge resorption can be devastating.

Let me be clear that I do not have a big secret or magic bullet for atraumatic extraction. Instead I have curated many small secrets and tips that together result in a very comfortable, atraumatic, and ridge-preserving experience for the extraction patient. I call this technique the *atraumatic extraction technique* (*AET*). The goal of the AET is to preserve the patient's original jaw anatomy as much as possible and therefore preserve their facial structure.

Root Space Creation Extraction Technique

One of the major components of the AET is the root space creation extraction technique (RSCET). With this technique, root structure is removed to allow space for the remaining tooth structure to be pressured into prior to its removal, thereby preventing the need for bone removal and protecting the socket from deformation.

Why not remove tooth structure that will already be removed instead of removing bone to make the space needed to extract the tooth? Bone is difficult to replace once it's gone, but the tooth is coming out anyway, so it can be sacrificed during the extraction process.

Also, removing bone between the roots of multirooted teeth to allow space for further root and tooth removal is not as damaging as removing socket wall bone for the same ends.[7] Bone removed between roots will regenerate as the socket heals, but socket wall bone will heal by resorbing toward the center of ridge, resulting in a narrower ridge.[7]

Roots can be more easily removed when the periodontal ligament is severed and a space is created to move the root into. Prying a root out only increases the risk of root fracture and damage to the socket wall.[8,9] The RSCET therefore entails vertical sectioning of the root. When you remove some root structure vertically all the way through the apex, you can push the root laterally into this space (Fig 1-2), thereby facilitating removal without damaging the socket wall or alveolar ridge. If one vertical cut is not adequate to allow lateral movement of the root, then the root should be cut into four pieces with two vertical cuts at 90 degrees to each other.

When sectioning the root vertically, it is important to cut entirely through the apex; otherwise, when you apply pressure between the roots laterally, you may fracture the root above the apex, leaving the apex connected to one of the root pieces (Fig 1-3). If this occurs, sectioning should continue all the way through the apex, and the root remnant can be removed along with the other half of the root.

The rest of this book covers the basic AET, which includes the RSCET. These techniques can be applied to all extraction situations. However, each area of the mouth has specific characteristics that must be considered to help prevent extractions from becoming an exercise in frustration. After all, when extractions become excessively time-consuming, poor healing and complications result.[1] As such, subsequent chapters address specific teeth and areas of the mouth to maximize success with the AET and RSCET.

Conclusion

Extractions can be very traumatic and damaging to the oral anatomy. Forceps are designed to luxate teeth either by rotation or buccolingual movement, which can damage the buccal, lingual, mesial, and distal socket walls. Elevators use lateral leverage and wedging forces, causing trauma to hard and soft tissues.

If a traumatic extraction occurs, the result is resorption of the buccal and lingual bony walls, restriction of blood supply, and increased inflammation.[2,3,5] Without socket preservation, there is an average of 4.5 mm of horizontal bone resorption and 1.5 mm of vertical bone resorption within the first 6 months.[3,10–12]

After extraction, the buccal ridge exhibits more resorption than the lingual ridge.[7] This can influence implant placement, shifting the implant position more lingual and therefore requiring a restoration with a buccal cantilever or an inadequate occlusal table.

This is why an atraumatic extraction technique with socket preservation is so important—because it helps reduce buccal ridge resorption and thereby protects the patient's original jaw anatomy and facial structure. This book will show you how.

References

1. Laskin DM. Oral and Maxillofacial Surgery. St Louis: Mosby, 1980.
2. Borle RM. Textbook of Oral and Maxillofacial Surgery. New Delhi: JP Medical, 2014.
3. Jambhekar S, Kermen F, Bidra AS. Clinical and histologic outcomes of socket grafting after flapless tooth extraction: A systematic review of randomized controlled clinical trials. J Prosthet Dent 2015;113:371–382.
4. Zafiropoulos GG, Kasaj HA, Hoffman O. Immediate implant placement in fresh mandibular molar extraction socket: 8-year results. A case report. J Oral Implantol 2010;36:145–151.
5. Albeshri S, Greenstein G. Significance of facial bone thickness after dental implantations in healed ridges: A literature review. Compend Contin Educ Dent 2021;42:528–535.
6. Misawa M, Lindhe M, Araújo MG. The alveolar process following single-tooth extraction: A study of maxillary incisor and premolar sites in man. Clin Oral Implants Res 2016;27:884–889.
7. El-Chaar ES. Immediate placement and provisionalization of implant-supported, single-tooth restorations: A retrospective study. Int J Periodontics Restorative Dent 2011;31:409–419.
8. Hupp JR, Ellis E, Tucker MR. Contemporary Oral and Maxillofacial Surgery, ed 5. St Louis: Mosby, 2008:185–199.
9. Mehra P, D'Innocenzo R. Manual of Minor Oral Surgery for the General Dentist, ed 2. Hoboken: Wiley, 2016
10. Lekovic V, Kenny EB, Weinlaender M, et al. A bone regenerative approach to alveolar ridge maintenance following tooth extraction. Report of 10 cases. J Periodontol 1997;68:563–570.
11. Lekovic V, Camargo PM, Klokkevold PR, et al. Preservation of alveolar bone in extraction sockets using bioabsorbable membranes. J Periodontol 1998;69:1044–1049.
12. Iasella JM, Greenwell H, Miller RL, et al. Ridge preservation with freeze-dried bone allograft and a collagen membrane compared to extraction alone for implant site development: A clinical and histologic study in humans. J Periodontol 2003;74:990–999.

2

General Principles of the Atraumatic Extraction Technique

At some point in our lives, we have all been advised not to "sweat the small stuff." I'm telling you the opposite. In the world of atraumatic extractions, paying attention to the small stuff is literally what saves bone and makes the experience better for the patient. Contrary to what some believe, tooth extraction is not a race. I have heard others brag that they "extracted 6 teeth in 6 minutes." Okay, but at what long-term cost to the patient? The bone lost due to the trauma of a forceful extraction may never be able to be fully regained.

Successful extraction is the combination of many careful and atraumatic steps that result in an atraumatic procedure. It's not about just one fancy technique or instrument. As such, the atraumatic extraction technique (AET) can be distilled into the following principles:

1. Develop a plan.
2. Take your time (plan the path of removal).
3. Administer slow, gentle anesthesia.
4. Perform minimal or no soft tissue reflection.
5. Divide and conquer (between roots and within the roots themselves, using the root space creation extraction technique [RSCET]).

Preoperative Evaluation

The preoperative evaluation must include a thorough review of the patient's medical history, including any medications they have taken or are currently taking and with particular attention for any use of anticoagulants or the presence of hypertension or osteoporosis. Bone may fracture more easily in patients with reduced blood supply or brittle bone (ie, in the case of osteoporosis).

The patient's psychologic and emotional state must also be considered. Is the patient anxious? Is sedation necessary? What is their dental treatment history? Do they have any previous negative experience with extractions? Do they have a past history of difficult anesthesia? Does it wear off quickly? **Listen and believe patients** when they tell you that anesthesia wears off quickly for them or that they have had a bad experience with a previous extraction. Ask what it was about the extraction that bothered them. Was it the noises, smells, or bedside manner of the clinician? Any of this information can be used to adjust the environment for the patient at their appointment with you to increase their comfort level (and thereby the chances of a successful visit). If the patient feels heard and that their concerns were believed and addressed, they will undoubtedly return to you for further treatment and refer others to your practice.

Planning

Always have a game plan. A few moments of planning will prevent a long and stressful appointment. Visualize how you will remove the tooth or teeth with the least amount of trauma. Study the root form and shape of each tooth to be removed. Is it tapered, bulbous, or parallel-sided? Are there adjacent structures to be considered during removal, like nerves, bony structures, teeth, or restorations? If the root is tapered and narrower apically than coronally, severing the periodontal ligament fibers will facilitate extraction.

Is the width of the periodontal ligament narrow? If so, this could signify ankylosis. Percussion with a resultant hollow sound may also indicate ankylosis. If root resorption is present, then the chances of ankylosis are much greater, and the tooth should be assumed to be ankylosed.

Is it possible to expand the socket with minimal damage to the bone? The mandibular alveolar bone is denser than that of the maxilla, so it is easier to expand maxillary sockets. If extracting multiple teeth, an elevator should be used between them to luxate each against the other to obtain initial mobility.

Never assume that any extraction will be "easy." Teeth are designed to stay in place!

Tooth access for extraction

There are two categories of access: general access to the mouth and access to the tooth or teeth being treated. Where in the mouth is the tooth requiring extraction? Does the patient have difficulty opening? Do they gag? Are adjacent teeth close and vulnerable to damage during the procedure? Are there restorations on adjacent teeth that may be dislodged during the extraction procedure?

Surgical assistant's role

The surgical assistant is vital to success with the AET. Their primary responsibilities are maintaining suction for clear visibility and patient comfort, preparing the instrument tray with instruments ready in the predetermined order, and placing the bite block to stabilize the mandible. The bite block protects the patient's temporomandibular joint (TMJ) from damage, resists any forces generated during the extraction, takes pressure off the masticatory muscles required in opening and thereby minimizes muscle fatigue, and of course frees up the assistant to help during the procedure itself. However, because the patient will be unable to swallow with the bite block in place, the surgical assistant must keep the oral cavity clear of fluids. Note that the bite block needs to be removed periodically to allow the patient to swallow and the mouth to be rinsed out.

Tooth factors to consider

The following factors specific to the tooth or teeth to be extracted must be considered in the course of planning the extraction.

Condition of crown

Is there a full-coverage restoration? Is there an endodontic access opening? Is there a large amalgam restoration with minimal tooth structure? Is the tooth fractured with no restoration? All of these considerations will impact the path of removal planned.

Condition of root

Has the tooth been treated with endodontics? Endodontic treatment results in more brittle roots, vulnerable to fracture. Are there resorption lesions present? Is there subgingival decay so that the crown breaks off or comes off easily?

Mobility of tooth

Is there any bone loss evident from evaluating the crown-root ratio? If so, is the bone loss vertical or horizontal? A widened periodontal ligament space signifies increased mobility.

Radiographic evaluation

What is the relationship of the roots to the vital structures, including the mandibular canal, maxillary sinus, nasal floor, incisive foramen, mental foramen, and adjacent teeth? What is the configuration of the roots? Are they bulbous or dilacerated (which could inhibit removal in the long axis of the socket)? Are they narrow or fractured? Weak points prone to fracture, such as at the ends of posts, which are points of concentration of stress, should be identified prior to the procedure. Maxillary bone is more porous, while mandibular bone is denser, meaning that there is much higher chance of root fracture in the mandible versus the maxilla. A lone-standing tooth—versus a span of teeth—has more of a tendency to come out with some bone attached because the remainder of the ridge is resorbed and narrower.

Approach tooth removal carefully, being sure to minimize stress to any adjacent teeth and bony structures.

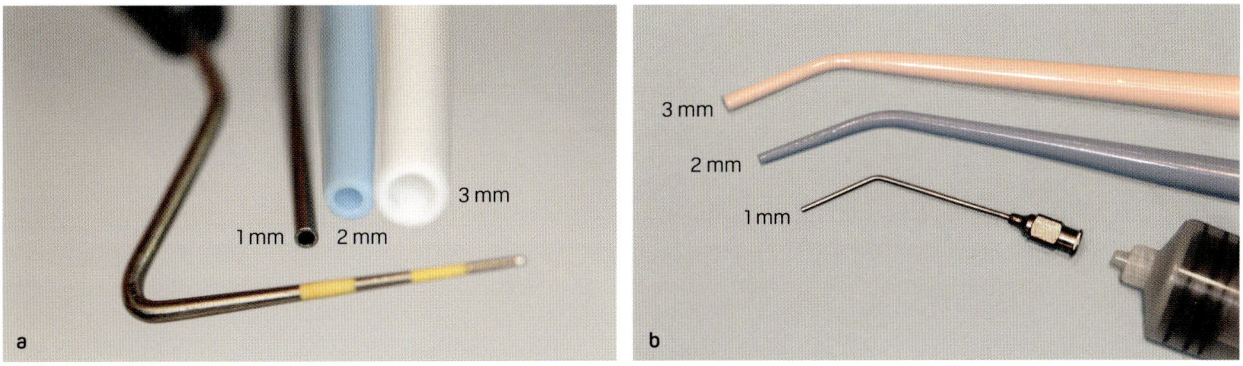

FIG 2-1 *(a and b)* Small and medium suction tip sizes and irrigation syringe with thin tip.

Instruments to use

Forceps, elevators, and periotomes need to be sharp to be effective. Irrigation syringes with thin tips should be used with two different sizes of suction tips: small and medium (Fig 2-1). The medium tips are indicated for general use during most of the extraction procedure. The small suction tips are helpful to improve vision in vertical cuts on roots by removing tooth debris during irrigation in these areas.

THE GREETER DOGS IN MY OFFICE

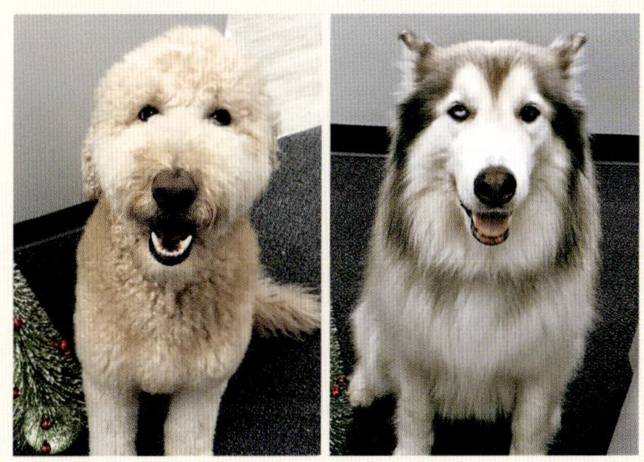

Gibbs Micco

Anesthesia and Patient Management

The first of many steps in a successful atraumatic extraction and successful socket preservation is gentle, atraumatic anesthesia. Also central to a successful appointment is proper patient management.

During the appointment, project a relaxed vibe so the patient feels at ease. Provide the patient sunglasses to dim the harsh overhead fluorescent lights, headphones to mask any procedure noises (possibly with their own music), and a soft blanket to keep them warm and comfortable in the often-cold dental chair and office. All of this combines to help settle the patient down, similar to swaddling a baby or getting cozy before going to bed, but it also indicates that you care about them and their comfort.

For many patients, the presence of well-behaved dogs in the office can also help to relax them. Petting a dog is naturally relaxing for most people, and it reduces blood pressure and takes the patient's mind off the upcoming procedure.

Masking certain words that instill fear or panic will help to keep your patient relaxed during the procedure. Therefore, consider using the following terms during conversation in the presence of patients:

- "end" for needle
- "s" for scissors
- "color" for blood
- "12" or "15" for scalpel blade

Make up your own vocabulary for dental terms that you perceive may cause anxiety in your patients.

Follow-Up Care

Part of the total package of the AET is calling to check on the patient the evening of the procedure. Not only will this show the patient that you care about them, but I have also noticed that patients are more likely to read through the aftercare instructions after they answer the phone. They want to be a "good patient" and heal well for you, and I believe patients heal more quickly when they know you care about them.

3

Atraumatic Anesthesia

"I'm real numb, Doc!"

There is an art to anesthesia administration. When I was a junior in dental school, on my oral surgery rotation, it was easy to spot the difference between the dental students, who pumped one carpule after another into their patients, and the chief resident, who was deliberate and measured, slowly adding anesthesia and allowing the tissue to absorb the fluid as he made conversation with the patient. The goal of anesthesia administration is not just a numb patient but a comfortable patient who feels like they are in control of the procedure.

Preparing the Patient

At the consult appointment before the procedure, it should be made clear to the patient that they will be in control during the entire procedure. Promises to deliver gentle anesthesia are important, but even more important are promises to halt the procedure if they feel anything. The patient needs to know and believe that they are in control and that if they tell you they are uncomfortable, you will not proceed until their comfort is addressed. Furthermore, you can apply some topical anesthetic at the end of this consult appointment to let them experience how powerful it is. Be calm and confident, and reassure them that they will be comfortable. Reassure them that you will not proceed if they feel any pain and that all they have to do is let you know—they are in control.

Preoperative medication

Lorazepam (Ativan, Pfizer) should be prescribed prior to the procedure to help the patient relax. The patient should take one 0.5- to 1.0-mg tablet the night before the appointment and another tablet 2 hours before the appointment. If the patient is still anxious when they arrive for the appointment, they can take a third tablet then. Ativan takes approximately 2 hours to take effect, so this three-dose regimen should do the trick.

Anesthetic Techniques

The recommendations and guidelines that follow in this chapter apply to adults. The practitioner must determine the maximum anesthetic volume on a case-by-case basis based on patient weight and other factors.

Before the patient enters the operatory, all instruments should be covered with a patient bib. Shiny instruments only create more anxiety in patients, and there is no need for the patient to see them.

At the beginning of the appointment and throughout, apply Aquaphor lubricant (Beiersdorf) to the patient's lips to ensure that gloves and instruments do not abrade them. Try to limit contact of the cold stainless steel instruments with the patient's lips and cheeks before the anesthesia has taken effect; this can be alarming and cause more anxiety in patients.

Maxillary Buccal Infiltration

First dry the buccal vestibule at the injection site. Apply topical anesthetic and wait 2 minutes, then dry the area and apply some more. Wait 30 seconds, then pull the buccal mucosa taught with dry gauze or mirror and **pull the tissue onto the needle**. A 30-gauge short needle should be used, and I advise using a less acidic anesthetic like mepivacaine HCl (Polocaine, Fresenius Kabi) or prilocaine HCl (Citanest Plain, AstraZeneca) first to reduce the "burn" patients feel. Inject about

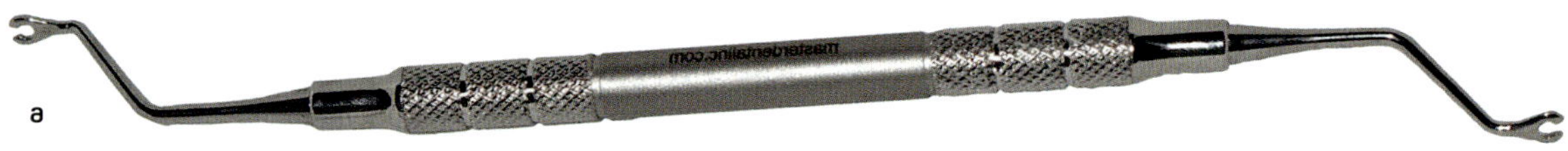

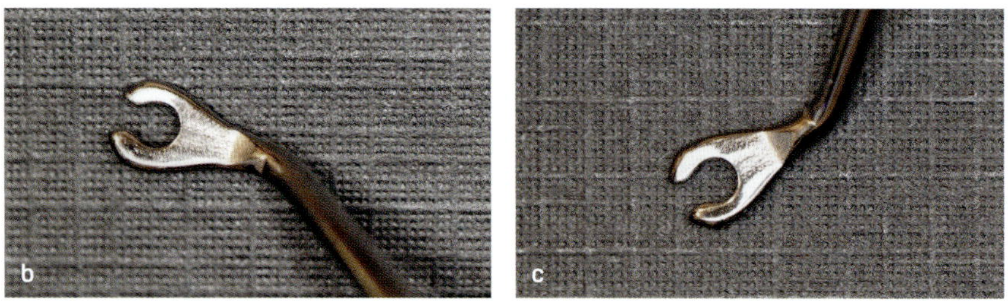

FIG 3-1 *(a)* The PAD is a double-ended stainless steel instrument with C-shaped ends. It is used to create a distraction and pressure anesthesia as the needle is inserted into the palatal tissue. *(b)* C-shaped end used for left palatal injections. *(c)* C-shaped end used for right palatal injections.

0.5 mL of mepivacaine HCl or prilocaine HCl without vasoconstrictor slowly, and then aspirate. Wait 30 to 60 seconds, and then inject 2% lidocaine HCl or 4% articaine (Septocaine, Henry Schein). Massage the area to distribute the anesthetic and force it deeper into the tissue.

It is important to release tension on the tissue after the needle is inserted so that it can accept anesthetic fluid without pressure, which will reduce discomfort for the patient. Talk the patient through the anesthetizing procedure, and reassure them that you will go slowly and gently. Wait for the anesthetic to take hold before continuing with the procedure.

Palatal Injections

The PAD

When I was 15 years old, I had my maxillary third molars removed. No sedation was prescribed, and I still remember the surprise and burning pain of the palatal injections. I literally rose out of the chair because it hurt so much. The palatal injections were fast and aggressive and administered without any warning. It was the worst part of the procedure by far—and the teeth were palatally impacted and difficult to remove.

As I progressed through my dental education and had to learn how to administer palatal injections myself, I was determined to find a way to anesthetize the palate more comfortably to protect my patients from the pain I once felt. There were many techniques described at the time, such as pressuring the palate with a mirror handle or cotton tip and injecting next to it. I decided I could do better. This led to the development of the patented PAD, or palatal anesthesia device[1,2] (Fig 3-1; available at masterdentalonline.com).

The PAD uses the principle of pressure anesthesia and the gate control theory of pain to alleviate the pain associated with a palatal injection. The stimulation of the surface tactile receptors by the instrument "opens the gate" of the pain-transmitting fibers and interrupts their transmission to the brain. (This is why you automatically rub your elbow when you bump it. Stimulating the surface tactile receptors blocks the pain pathway.) When the PAD is used to stimulate these surface receptors, the pain associated with the initial needle penetration is greatly reduced.

If you know the palatal injection will be painful, your body language and unease will convey that to the patient. The patient will sense it and anticipate a painful injection, which will only make the discomfort worse. On the other hand, when you know the palatal injection will be comfortable, your confidence and body language will convey that to the patient, and they will anticipate and experience a comfortable palatal injection.

The PAD has been shown to be vastly superior to conventional methods of palatal anesthesia through controlled clinical trials.[1] You will find this instrument to be a much more comfortable means of delivering palatal anesthesia. If you have been avoiding giving palatal anesthesia, it could be because your technique does not address adequate pain control. After all, pain control is just as important for the practitioner as it is for the patient.

Note: The PAD is used to apply pressure anesthesia and distraction to the palate prior to and during needle

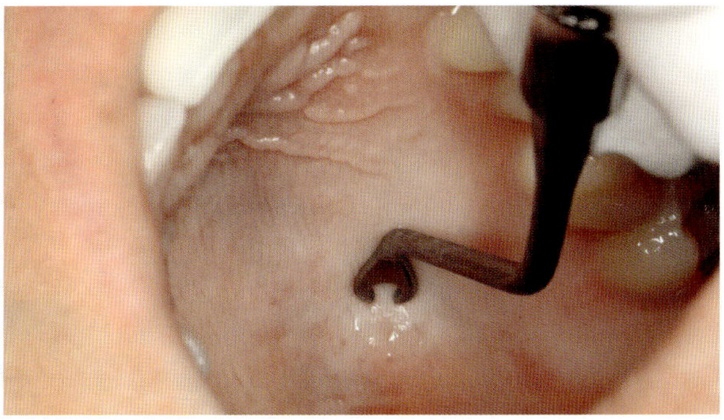

FIG 3-2 PAD used to apply pressure anesthesia and distraction to the left palate prior to needle insertion. The PAD is used to create pressure anesthesia and distraction *only* during needle insertion.

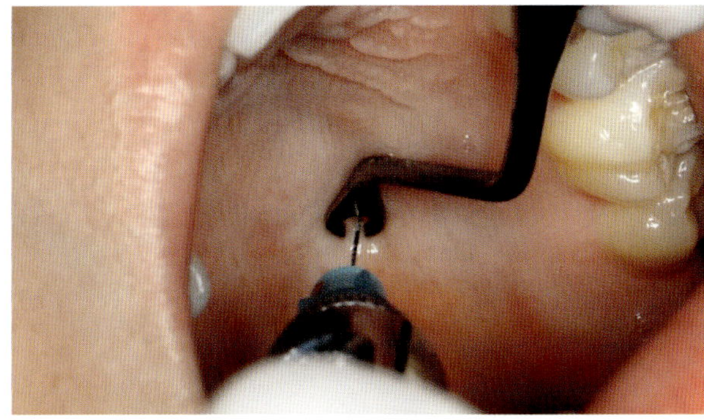

FIG 3-3 The needle is inserted immediately after the PAD is used to apply pressure to the palatal tissue. The PAD is then removed, and anesthetic is slowly injected. *The PAD is not used to apply pressure to the tissue as anesthetic is injected.*

insertion (Fig 3-2). It should not be used during injection of the anesthetic (Fig 3-3).

Palatal injection technique

First dry the palatal injection site. Apply topical anesthetic, and wait 2 minutes. Be sure to prevent the topical agent from running down the patient's throat, as this may cause gagging. Dry the area again and apply more topical anesthetic. Wait 30 seconds, and then place the right or left C-shaped end of the PAD on the palate. Inform the patient that they will feel some pressure. *Do not tell them they will feel a "pinch" or a "prick" because their body will feel what you told them it will.* Apply firm pressure with the C-shaped end to cause visible tissue blanching, and then insert the needle a few millimeters into the tissue. Withdraw the PAD, and then slowly inject anesthetic 0.1 mL at a time to blanch the tissue. Withdraw the needle, firmly rub the injection site, and then inject a few more increments of 0.1 mL anesthetic. Wait 2 minutes, then inject 2% lidocaine HCl or 4% articaine (Septocaine). This technique will result in a comfortable palatal injection primarily because you, as the one administering the anesthetic, have confidence that it will be comfortable.

Next, infiltrate in the vestibule, attached gingiva, papilla, and into the periodontal ligament space, especially on the lingual. Probe to confirm profound anesthesia. The patient should not be able to feel any pain; if they can, it will be more difficult to anesthetize during the procedure because they now have heightened anxiety. The patient may even perceive pressure or vibration as pain.

LONG-LASTING ANESTHESIA

I believe it is important to make sure our patients have anesthesia that lasts for an extended period of time following the procedure. I recommend the use of the long-lasting anesthetic bupivacaine HCl 0.5% (Marcaine, Pfizer) with 1:200,000 epinephrine, which lasts up to 7 hours. Up to two carpules can be injected per surgical site depending on patient age and weight. When using bupivacaine, there is a period of analgesia that persists after return of sensation; during this time, the need for strong analgesics is reduced. This helps our patients use fewer analgesics postsurgically. Also, if they have a long drive home, they are anesthetized all the way until they return home. When the procedure is completed, they are "waiting for the pain to begin." When they have prolonged anesthesia followed by analgesia, their anxiety decreases regarding postsurgical pain.

I recommend buccal infiltration of 0.5% bupivacaine HCl into the maxilla and mandible approximately 15 minutes into the procedure. (Note that bupivacaine is not indicated for nerve blocks.) If you administer bupivacaine early in the procedure, it is easier to maintain complete anesthesia during the procedure, and you will end up using less total anesthetic volume. This results in cost savings and less risk to the patient due to the reduced volume of anesthetic used.

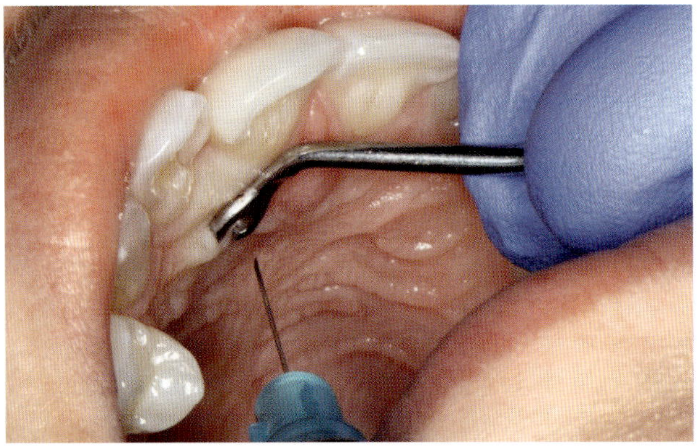

FIG 3-4 PAD used for an incisive injection.

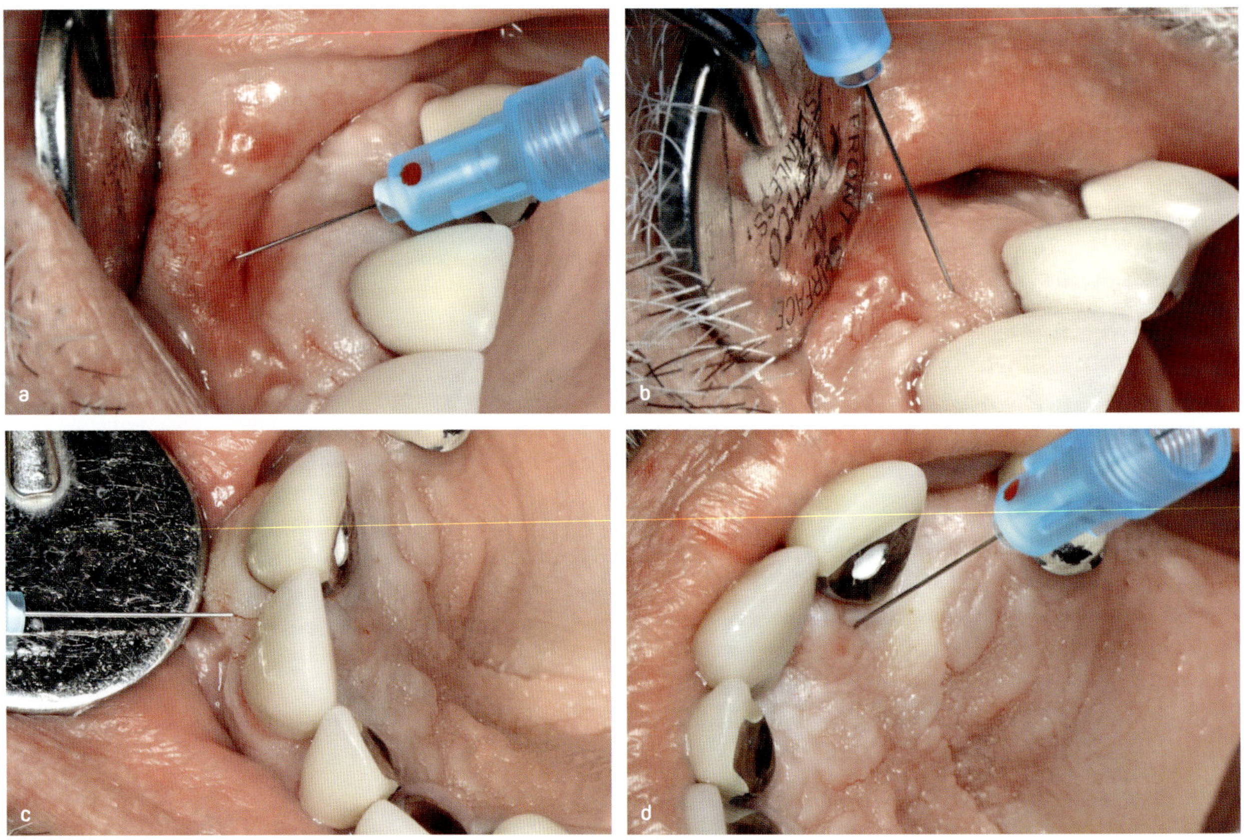

FIG 3-5 Incisive injection technique. *(a)* First anesthetize the facial of the maxillary central incisors, making sure to pull the tissue onto the needle. *(b)* Then use a 30-gauge needle to inject 3% mepivacaine HCl (Polocaine) without vasoconstrictor or 4% prilocaine HCl (Citanest Plain) horizontally at the facial into the base of the papilla between the central incisors. *(c)* Slowly move the needle palatally until the palatal surface of the papilla blanches. *(d)* Articaine 4% being injected next to the incisive papilla.

Incisive injection technique

While the PAD can be used for an incisive injection (Fig 3-4), I believe there is a more comfortable technique.

First anesthetize the facial of the maxillary central incisors using the anesthetic technique described above (Fig 3-5a). Then use a 30-gauge needle to inject 3% mepivacaine HCl (Polocaine) without vasoconstrictor or 4% prilocaine HCl (Citanest Plain) horizontally at the facial into the base of the papilla between the central incisors. Follow up with 2% lidocaine HCl or 4% articaine (Septocaine; Fig 3-5b). Slowly move the needle palatally until the palatal surface of the papilla blanches (Fig 3-5c). Finally, inject the same anesthetic into the palatal surface of the incisive papilla. Follow that with articaine next to the incisive papilla (Fig 3-5d). This technique will give adequate anesthesia to the palatal of the central incisors and may extend all the way to the palatal of the canines as well.

Mandibular Block

Dry the tissue and apply topical anesthetic twice during a 2-minute period. Using your thumb and dry gauze, stretch the tissue back to expose the injection site. Then use a 27-gauge to inject 2% lidocaine HCl into the site. (Note that 27-gauge needles are only used once for mandibular blocks because the bevel becomes bent and drags through tissue, which can lacerate tissues and vessels.) Insert the needle while jiggling the area with your thumb, and enter slowly. Then move the syringe toward the opposite side of the mouth to a position over the mandibular first molar. Aspirate repeatedly when injecting. Inject slowly while you talk to the patient; reassure them that they are doing great and ask them to take some slow breaths and to wiggle their toes (to help distract them).

Approximately 15 minutes into the procedure, add 0.5% bupivacaine by infiltration in the vestibule at the surgical site. Bupivacaine is not recommended to be used for a mandibular block injection. Infiltration in the buccal vestibule will keep the surgical area anesthetized for 5 to 7 hours, with analgesia that lasts a few hours. Generally, one to two carpules of bupivacaine per surgical site is sufficient depending on the size of the surgical site and the patient age and weight.

Postsurgical Medications

Methylprednisolone (Medrol Dosepak, Pfizer), a 6-day steroid regimen, should begin the day of the appointment. It should NOT be used in patients with diabetes, however, because it causes a rise in blood sugar. Ibuprofen 600 to 800 mg is also given at the time of the appointment to manage any immediate postoperative pain once the anesthesia wears off.

Postsurgically, a combination of 600 to 800 mg of ibuprofen and two 500-mg tablets of acetaminophen should be taken every 8 hours as needed for postoperative discomfort. Many studies confirm the effectiveness of this combination analgesic approach.[3]

INFECTION

Be aware that if infection is present, it may be difficult to anesthetize the patient due to the reduced pH in the tissues. In this case, you may need to wait slightly longer for the anesthesia to work.

Infection in the tissues causes production of acidic products, resulting in a reduction of the pH of the localized area.[2] The pH of normal healthy tissue is 7.4, but this is reduced to 5 to 6 when infection sets in.[2]

The pH of local anesthetics without vasoconstrictors is ~5.5, and anesthetics with vasoconstrictors have a pH of about 3.3 to 4.5. This is significant because the local anesthetics with vasoconstrictors "burn" more upon injection and have slower onset. Many factors contribute to this burning sensation: speed of injection, volume of solution delivered, temperature of the solution, density of the tissue, and the psychology of the situation. Nonetheless, local anesthetics without vasoconstrictors (ie, higher pH, less acidic) have quicker onset and are more comfortable for the patient upon injection.

References

1. Mason S. Comparison of the palatal anesthesia device (PAD) and the dental mirror handle (DMH) when used as pressure anesthesia of devices in decreasing the pain associated with needle insertion during a greater palatine nerve block [abstract]. Presented at the 81st General Session of the IADR, Göteborg, Sweden, June 2003.
2. Malamed SF. Handbook of Local Anesthesia, ed 4. St Louis: Mosby, 1997.
3. Daniels SE, Atkinson HC, Stanescu I, Frampton C. Analgesic efficacy of an acetaminophen/ibuprofen fixed-dose combination in moderate to severe postoperative dental pain: A randomized, double-blind, parallel-group, placebo-controlled trial. Clin Ther 2018;40: 1765–1776.e5.

4

Clinical Application of the Atraumatic Extraction Technique and Root Space Creation Extraction Technique

This chapter covers the basic atraumatic extraction technique (AET) using the root space creation extraction technique (RSCET). These techniques can be applied to all extraction situations where the teeth have minimal to no mobility and good bone support. (Teeth with Class II or Class III mobility can usually be removed atraumatically if there is adequate crown structure to grasp the tooth with a forceps.) Chapters 5 through 10 apply these techniques to specific teeth and areas of the mouth.

The RSCET involves using a bur to section vertically between multiple roots or within single roots and removing root structure to create a space into which roots (in multirooted teeth) or root halves (in single-rooted teeth) can be pressured so they can be mobilized and removed. If these roots or root halves cannot be removed in one piece, they can be sectioned again, and the remaining fragments can be pressured into the created space. This method of root removal is far less traumatic to the surrounding bone than traditional luxation with forceps—it preserves the bone by removing root structure instead of bone.

I believe these techniques are predictable methods for tooth extraction. They are not the quickest methods of removing teeth, but tooth extraction is not a race to be won. These techniques are more predictable and less traumatic than traditional methods, and that's what matters for the patient. (Note that certain situations may not require all of the steps to be followed; some may be deemed nonproductive or not applicable to the clinical situation and therefore can be skipped at the discretion of the operating dentist.)

Verify Profound Anesthesia

Probe the sulcus firmly with a periodontal probe and stimulate the adjacent gingiva, especially on the lingual, to confirm that you have profound anesthesia. If not, administer either another nerve block or infiltration. Articaine is most effective for infiltration, and it is helpful to infiltrate into the sulcus circumferentially.

A bite block can be used to stabilize the mandible; this also helps patients hold their mouths open during the procedure without making their muscles sore. This is especially important when working in the mandible, because pressure may be applied in a downward direction, stressing the masticatory muscles, but it is also useful when working in the maxilla to help prevent muscle fatigue.

Release Periodontal Ligament Fibers Without Flap Reflection

Using a thin periotome or a 12D scalpel blade, enter the sulcus by applying vertical pressure with a rocking motion (Fig 4-1a). Be careful not to apply too much pressure on the buccal or facial, because the bone is thin in these areas and is vulnerable to fracture. It may be helpful to use a scalpel blade first to excise some fibers and get a good start, and then reenter with the periotome. Use the periotome to excise fibers as deeply as possible, circling the tooth twice (Figs 4-1b and 4-1c).

You may find it difficult to get into the sulcus due to lack of space or ankylosis. If so, use a surgical-length

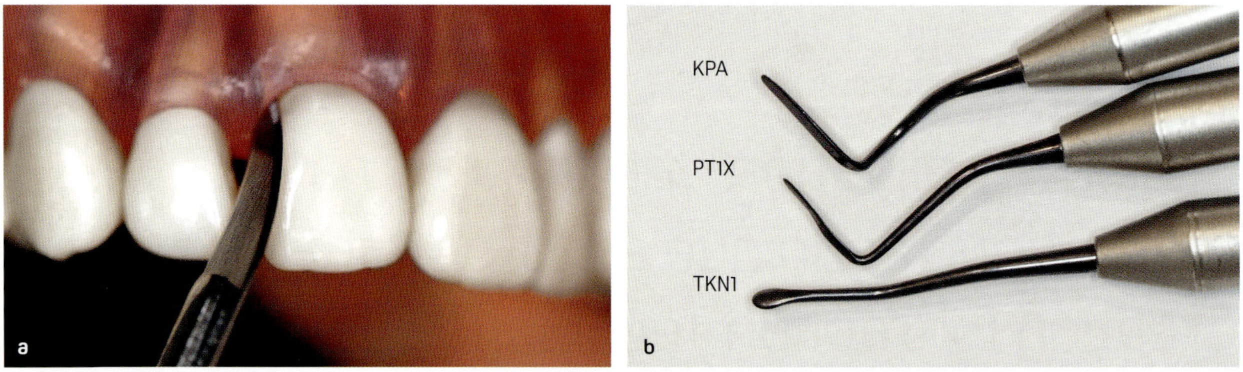

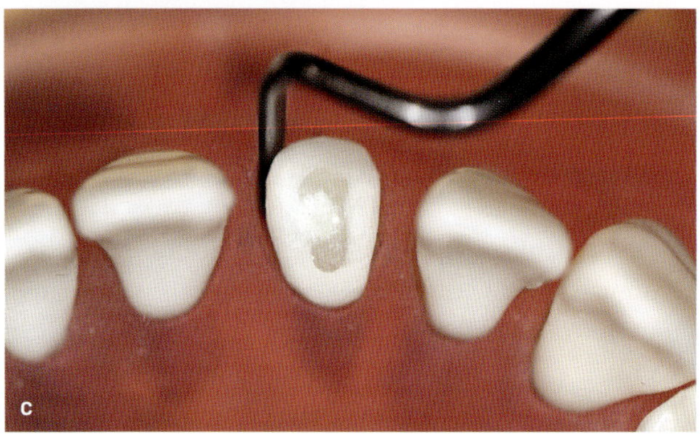

FIG 4-1 *(a)* A 12D scalpel blade is inserted into the distofacial sulcus of the maxillary right central incisor to release the periodontal ligament fibers by applying vertical pressure with a back-and-forth rocking motion. *(b)* Hu-Friedy periotomes. *(c)* Periotome in the sulcus using vertical pressure and a back-and-forth rocking motion.

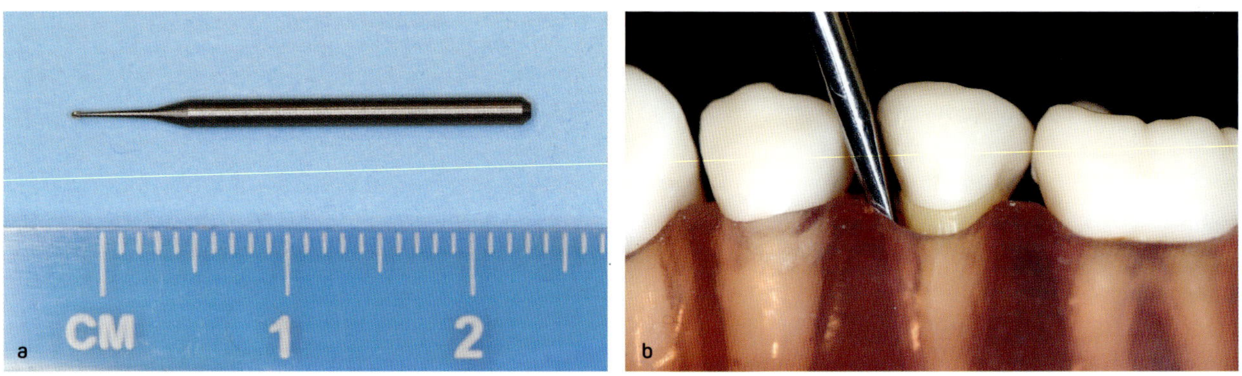

FIG 4-2 *(a)* Surgical-length ¼ round high-speed bur to enter the sulcus. *(b)* The bur is used in an up-and-down pumping motion to open the periodontal ligament space.

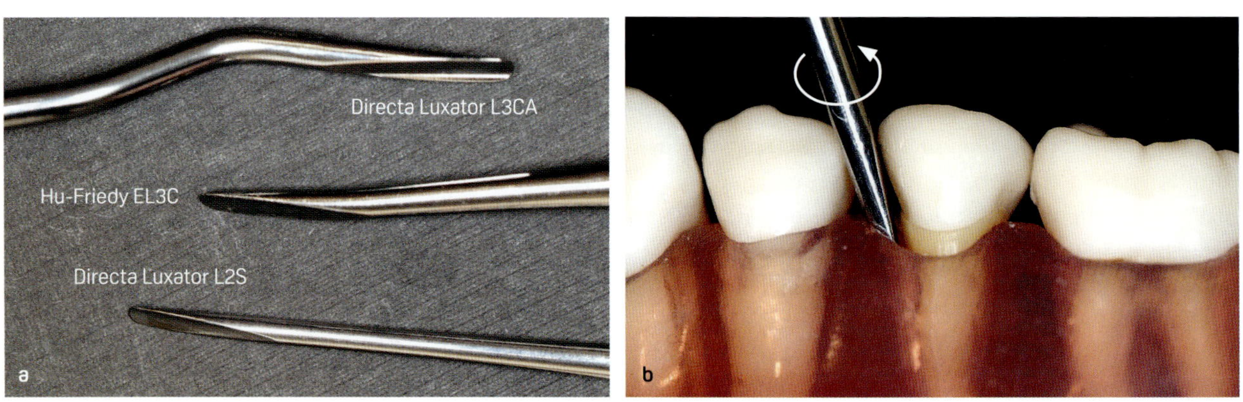

FIG 4-3 *(a)* Examples of thin elevators. *(b)* Directa Luxator L2S used in a twisting motion at the mesiobuccal of the mandibular left second premolar.

¼ round high-speed bur as follows (Fig 4-2): Use an up-and-down pumping motion at the mesial, distal, and lingual as deeply as possible. Try to cut in the direction of the root, not the socket wall. This opening of the periodontal ligament space releases the tooth from the adjacent bone, making it easier to remove, and forms a space for an elevator to enter and pressure the root. The periotome, scalpel, or round bur can be used in any order.

Attempt Tooth Removal Coronally Without Flap Reflection

Introduce a thin elevator at the mesiobuccal and distobuccal (Fig 4-3a), and use a twisting motion to attempt to move the tooth coronally (Fig 4-3b).

At this point, if the tooth cannot be mobilized with a thin elevator or if there is not enough crown present to luxate the tooth but the root is intact, you can use the Easy X-Trac System (A. Titan) or Benex Root Extraction System (Meisinger) (see chapter 12). This applies to all single roots or single-rooted teeth except the mandibular incisors (nos. 23–26). The mandibular incisors are generally too thin mesiodistally to be removed with Easy X Trac or Benex. Easy X-Trac and Benex both involve drilling a hole down the middle of the root into the root canal space and inserting a threaded rod. This rod is pulled coronally with a wedging device, removing the root in one piece. To accomplish this, the crown must be cut horizontally approximately 1 mm above the gingival margin, being aware of the gingival margin location to avoid lacerating the gingiva.

Reduce Interproximal Contacts; Luxate Gently with Forceps

The concept of atraumatic tooth removal pertains not only to the tooth being extracted but also to the adjacent teeth, their restorations, and the rest of the mouth as well. Therefore, it is important to reduce the interproximal contact surfaces on the tooth to be removed so that slight luxation does not move or harm adjacent teeth or restorations. Once that has been accomplished, place forceps as far apically as possible without engaging bone. Try to engage the root surface apical to any restoration margins. Gently apply pressure apically and hold for 30 seconds, then gently luxate using a rotational motion to test the mobility of the tooth. If the bone is thick on either the buccal or lingual, slight pressure can be placed in that direction. When pressure is applied coronally in a lateral direction, that pressure is felt cervically and apically (Fig 4-4).

If gentle luxation is not successful in removing the tooth, the crown should be sectioned horizontally about 1 mm coronal to the gingival margin, as described in the next section.

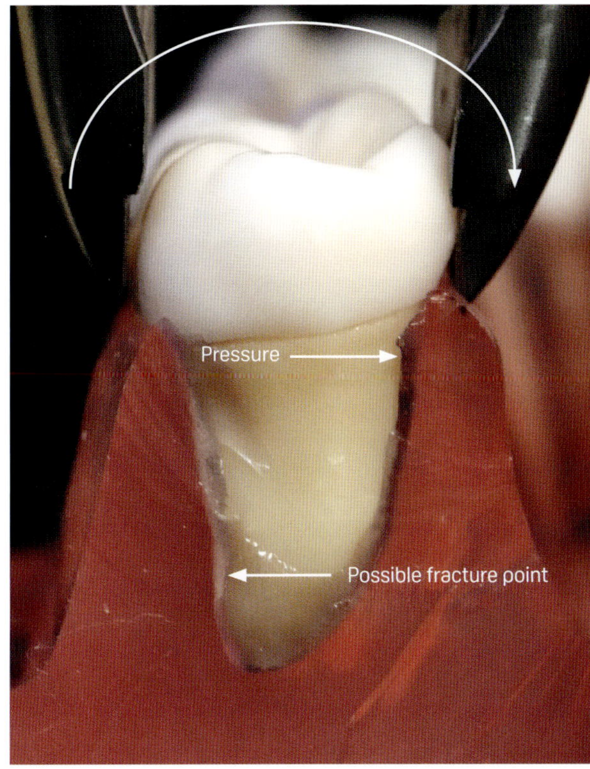

FIG 4-4 Pressure applied coronally toward the lingual with forceps on the mandibular left first molar. This also pressures the buccal surfaces of the mesial and distal roots, which may result in apical fracture.

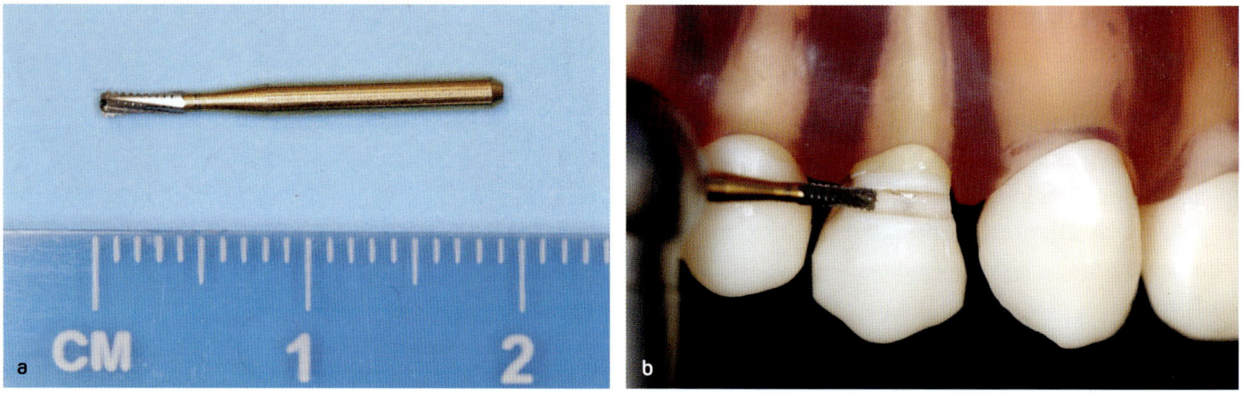

FIG 4-5 *(a)* Great White high-speed crosscut fissure bur. *(b)* The bur is used to horizontally section a maxillary right first premolar 1 mm coronal to the free gingival margin.

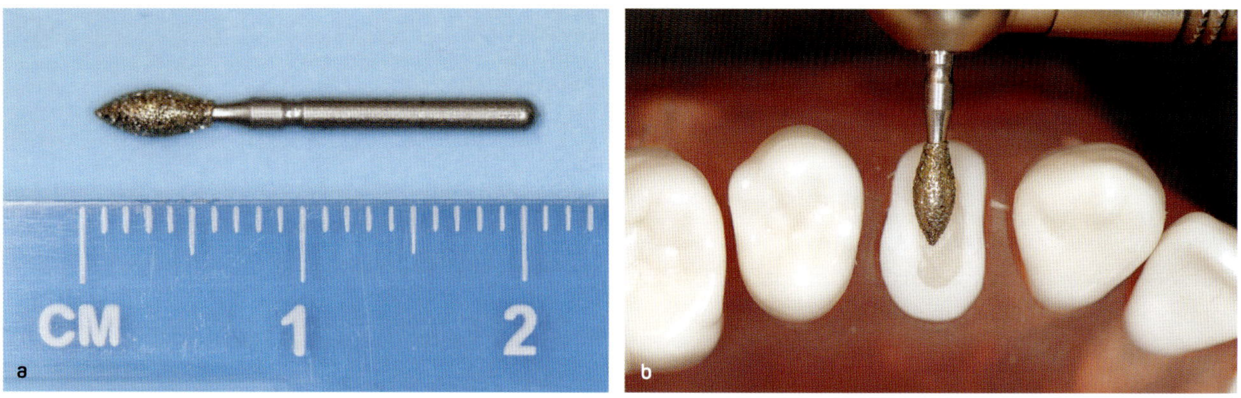

FIG 4-6 *(a)* High-speed football diamond bur. *(b)* After horizontally sectioning the crown, the bur is used to smooth the remaining tooth structure to a level 1 mm coronal to the free gingival margin.

Section Crown Horizontally at the Cementoenamel Junction

Some practitioners remove the crown as the first step in every extraction, feeling that it is the most efficient and atraumatic method.

When sectioning a crown or roots, it is important to use plenty of saline irrigation to remove tooth debris and to use a thin irrigation tip that will reach the apex of the roots you are sectioning. This allows you to see and feel in these areas.

Using a Great White high-speed crosscut fissure bur (SS White), section the crown 1 mm coronal to the gingival margin (Fig 4-5). It is important to be aware of the gingival margin location to avoid lacerating the gingiva. Section two-thirds of the way through the crown, and then, using an elevator, gently pry off the crown. Using a football-shaped diamond bur, smooth the remaining tooth structure to create a fairly flat surface (Fig 4-6). This allows you to see the remaining root structure anatomy and determine the best location to section. Vertical fractures may be evident also. Leaving the tooth 1 mm above the gingival margin allows a starting point for a thin elevator, a surgical-length ¼ round high-speed bur, or a periotome to enter the sulcus and pressure the root.

Multirooted Teeth

Section between roots; Elevate gently

Before sectioning, evaluate the radiographic appearance of roots to determine the depth of cut required to separate the roots. Use a surgical-length high-speed

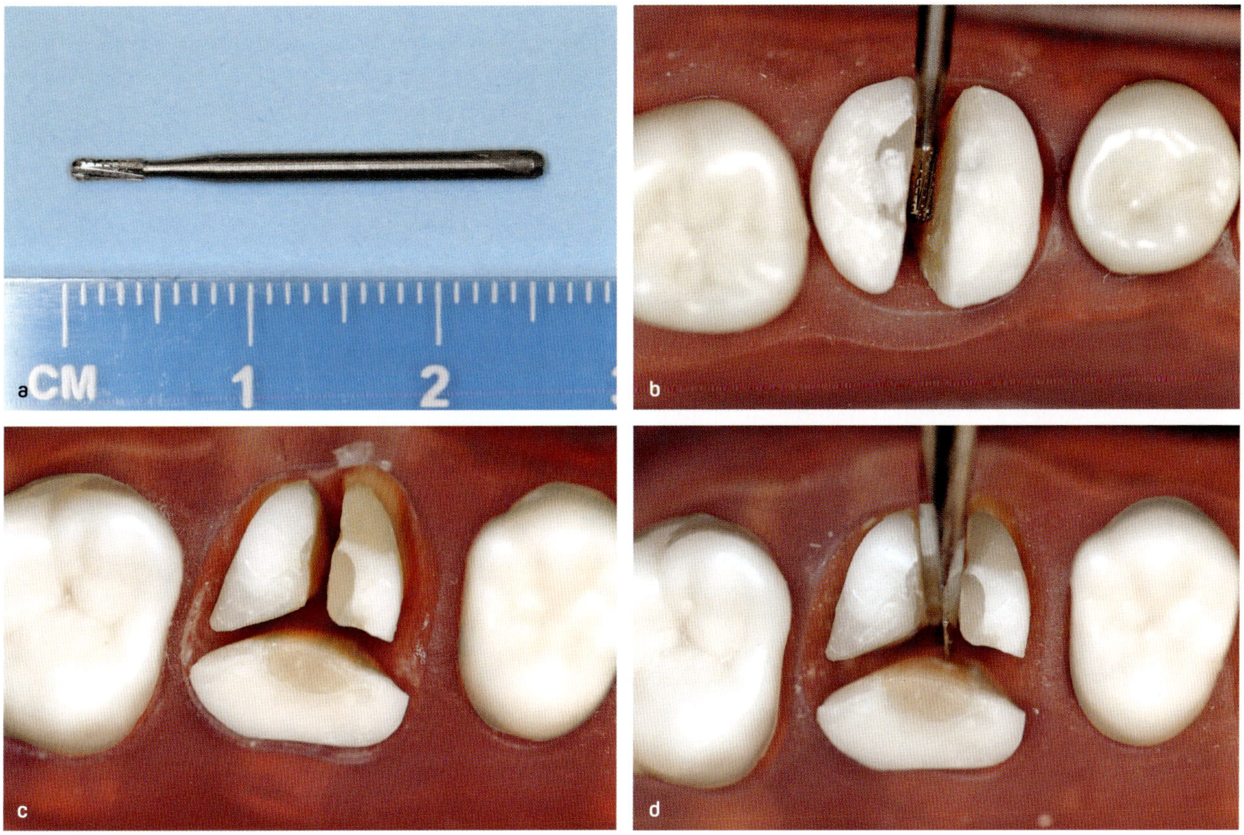

FIG 4-7 *(a)* Surgical-length high-speed crosscut fissure bur. *(b)* The bur is used to section a mandibular left first molar vertically in a buccolingual direction in the furcation between the mesial and distal roots. *(c)* A maxillary right first molar sectioned in a Y pattern, separating the mesiobuccal, distobuccal, and palatal roots. *(d)* An elevator is introduced between the roots and, using gentle rotation, pressures the roots laterally, taking care not to fracture the buccal or lingual bone.

crosscut fissure bur for this procedure (Fig 4-7a). For mandibular molars, section the mesial and distal roots in a buccolingual direction (Fig 4-7b). For maxillary molars, section in a Y pattern (Fig 4-7c). Introduce an elevator between the roots and, using gentle rotation, pressure the roots laterally (Fig 4-7d). Be careful not to fracture the buccal or lingual bone.

Enter sulcus laterally; Pressure roots into space

Using an Orban knife or a thin elevator, enter the sulcus on the lateral surfaces of the roots and attempt to force the roots into the space created by sectioning between the roots (Fig 4-8). Be aware that you are pressuring against the adjacent bone, so do this gently, paying attention to the adjacent bone. You may find that reentering and sectioning deeper between the roots is required.

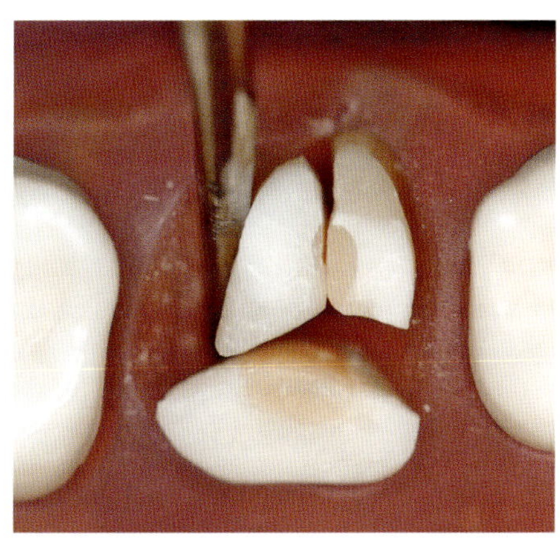

FIG 4-8 The distobuccal root is pressured mesially into the space created by separating roots.

Single-Rooted Teeth and Individual Roots of Multirooted Teeth

Release periodontal ligament fibers again; Attempt root removal coronally without flap reflection

Using the narrow periotome, enter the sulcus, applying vertical pressure and a back-and-forth rocking motion to excise the periodontal ligament fibers further apically. Introduce a thin elevator at the mesiobuccal and distobuccal, using a twisting motion to attempt to move the root coronally (Fig 4-9). If the root moves but not coronally, release the periodontal ligament fibers again with the periotome, then try the elevators again at the mesiobuccal and distobuccal. If you are not able to remove the roots at this point, the next step is to vertically section the roots themselves.

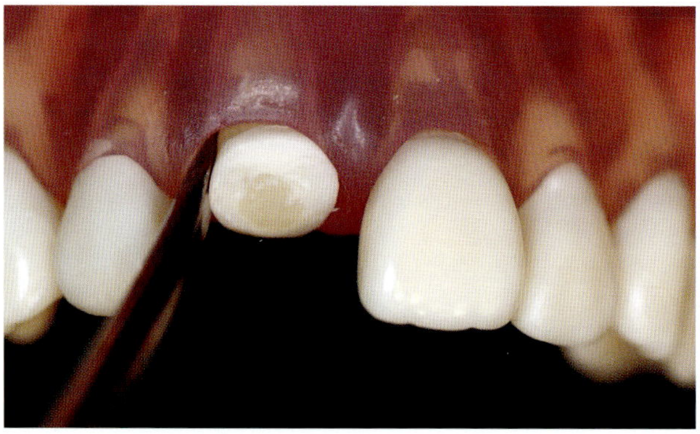

FIG 4-9 A thin elevator (Hu-Friedy EL3C) is used to gently luxate the root of a maxillary right central incisor with a twisting motion to elevate the root out of socket.

Section roots vertically; Elevate gently

Using the surgical-length high-speed crosscut fissure bur, section the roots vertically (Fig 4-10a). Section mandibular molar roots in a mesiodistal direction. Section maxillary molar buccal and palatal roots in a buccolingual direction. Section roots of single-rooted teeth in a buccolingual direction so that luxation does not stress the buccal bone.

It is very important to section all the way through the apex (see note below). If the surgical-length crosscut fissure bur does not reach the apex, use a straight handpiece bur to complete cutting through the apex (Fig 4-10b). This requires opening up the cut wider at the coronal aspect to allow room for the shank of the straight handpiece bur.

Introduce an elevator between the root sections and pressure them using gentle rotation (Fig 4-10c). Be careful not to fracture the buccal or lingual bone.

Note: If you do not section all the way through to the apex, luxating the two halves of the root will result in a fracture coronal to the apex, leaving a root tip in place. If this occurs, remove the loose root fragment (Fig 4-10d). The choice is then to attempt to pressure the remaining root into the space created by removing the root fragment, or to section through the apex.

Enter sulcus laterally; Pressure roots into space

Using an Orban knife or a thin elevator, enter the sulcus on the lateral surfaces of the roots and attempt to force the roots into the space created by sectioning roots (RSCET; Fig 4-11). Be aware that you are placing pressure against the adjacent bone, so do this in a gentle manner, paying attention to the adjacent bone. You may find that reentering and sectioning deeper between the roots is required. Entering the sectioned space with an elevator and pressuring the root fragments laterally also may be helpful. If this does not mobilize the root fragments, it may be necessary to section them again. This is generally more applicable to larger roots, but smaller roots also may require this step, at which time you will actually be drilling out the entire root. Again, it is necessary to drill through the apex; this is indicated by the feeling of the bur "dropping" into the softer bone.

If the root is moving laterally, but you cannot elevate it out, a helpful tip is to use a hemostat—not a rongeur because it is too stiff—and clamp as far apically as possible onto the sectioned root fragment. Then, move the hemostat back and forth slowly, applying constant pulling pressure and taking care not to break the root. As you slowly move back and forth, try to clamp deeper onto the root. Usually, you will be able to remove the root fragment in one piece (Fig 4-12).

Continue to elevate and remove sectioned root pieces, sectioning them into smaller pieces if needed. Once all root pieces are removed, proceed to socket debridement (see chapter 11).

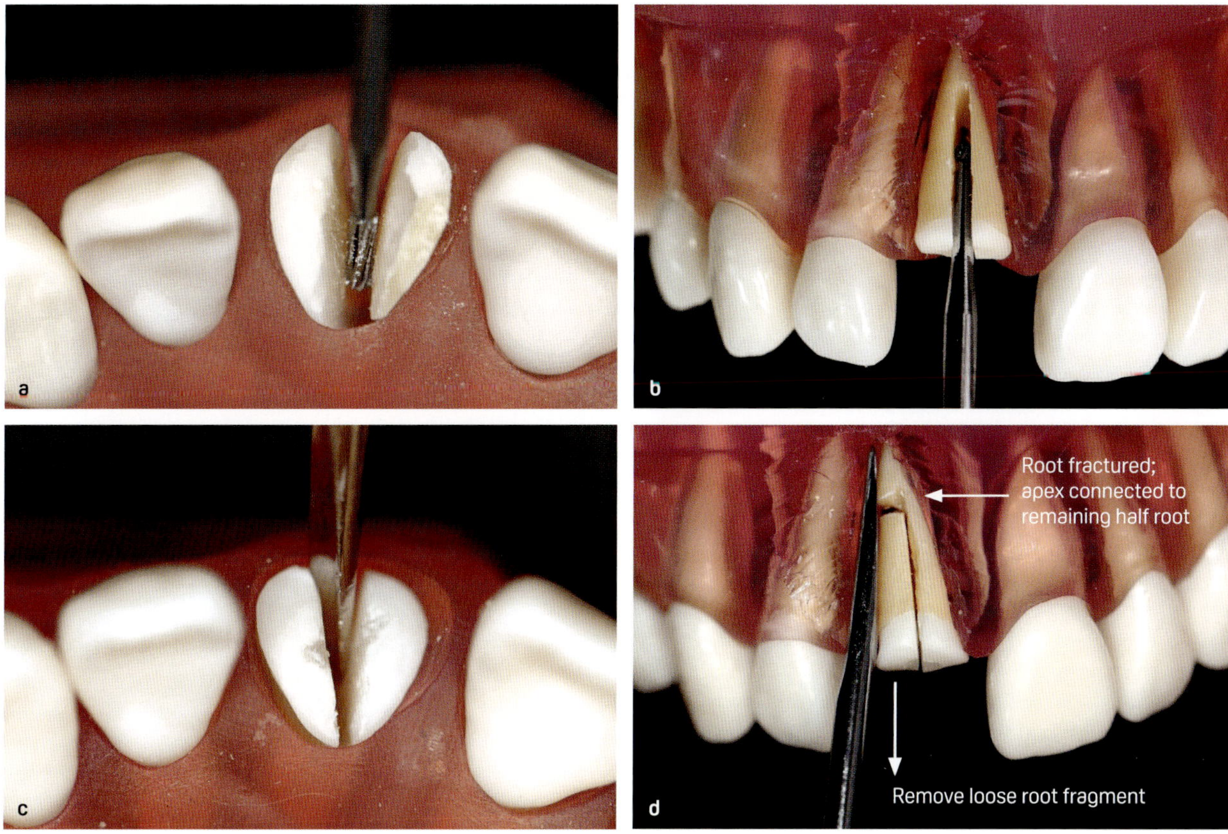

FIG 4-10 *(a)* A surgical-length high-speed crosscut fissure bur is used to create space into which the root halves can be pressured (RSCET). When you feel the bur "drop" into the softer bone, you know you have sectioned through the apex. Cut toward the lingual and facial slightly to make sure the cut is through the root structure. *(b)* If the surgical-length crosscut fissure bur does not reach the apex, use a #4 or #6 round straight handpiece bur to complete sectioning of the root by cutting through the apex into the soft bone underneath. *(c)* Pressure sectioned roots laterally using a twisting motion with a thin elevator (Directa L2S or Hu-Friedy EL3C). *(d)* A thin elevator was used to apply pressure from the sulcus to a root that was not completely sectioned through the apex. A fracture of the root resulted, and the apex was left behind.

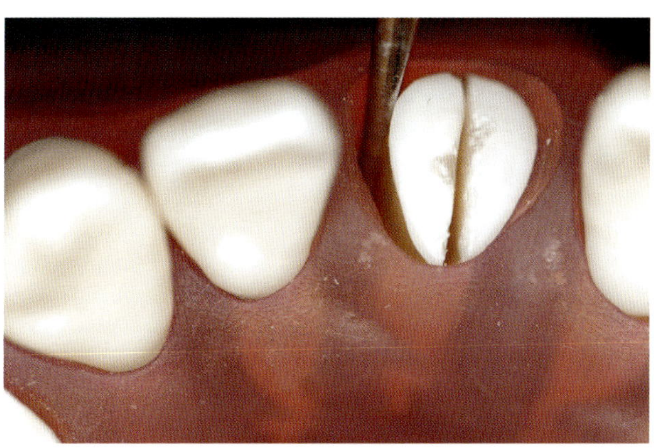

FIG 4-11 Using a Hu-Friedy Orban knife KO1/2IU, periotome, or thin elevator, enter the sulcus on the mesial and distal surfaces of the roots and attempt to force the roots into the space created by sectioning the roots (RSCET).

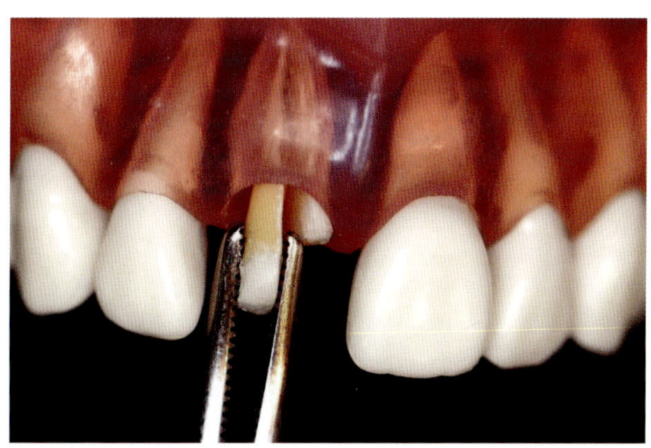

FIG 4-12 Root half mobilized by back-and-forth action of the hemostat as it is removed.

5

Atraumatic Extractions in the Anterior Maxilla: Find the Best Exit Route

The following atraumatic extraction techniques apply to maxillary canines and incisors with minimal to no mobility and good bone support. Obviously, teeth with Class II or III mobility can usually be removed atraumatically if there is adequate crown structure to grasp with a forceps. Also, it may not be necessary to use all of the following techniques to atraumatically remove a tooth. Some of the steps may be deemed nonproductive or not applicable to the clinical situation and therefore can be skipped at the discretion of the operating dentist.

The maxillary right central incisor is the demonstration example in this chapter; however, these principles apply to all maxillary canines and incisors since they have similarly shaped roots.

Verify Profound Anesthesia

Probe the sulcus with a periodontal probe and stimulate the adjacent gingiva, especially on the palatal, to confirm you have achieved profound anesthesia (Fig 5-1). If anesthesia is inadequate, administer either another nerve block or infiltration into the sulcus and adjacent vestibule or gingiva circumferentially (Fig 5-2). For quickest onset, use 4% articaine with 1:100,000 epinephrine. For hemostasis, 2% lidocaine 1:100,000 epinephrine is helpful.

A bite block can be used to stabilize the mandible; this also helps patients hold their mouth open during the procedure, reducing muscle fatigue.

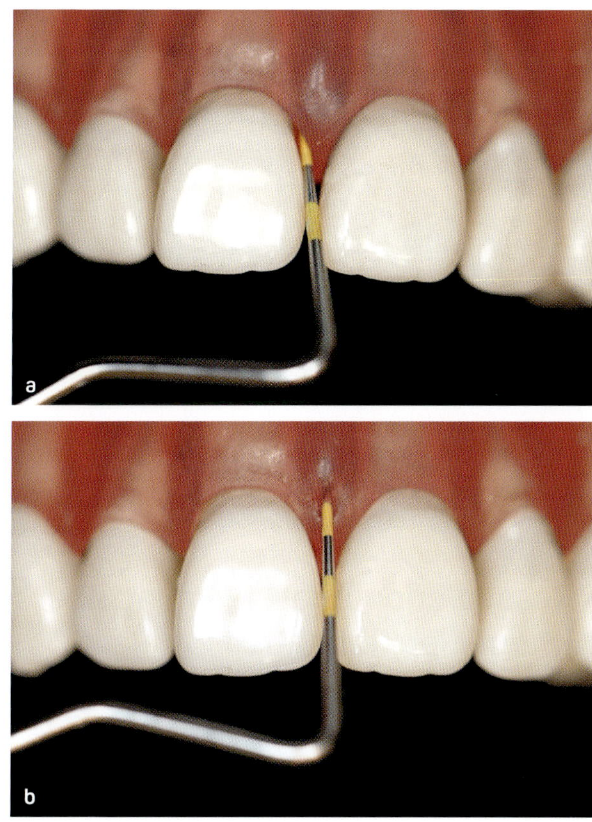

FIG 5-1 Verifying adequate anesthesia. *(a)* Probing the mesiofacial sulcus of the maxillary right central incisor. *(b)* Probing the gingiva.

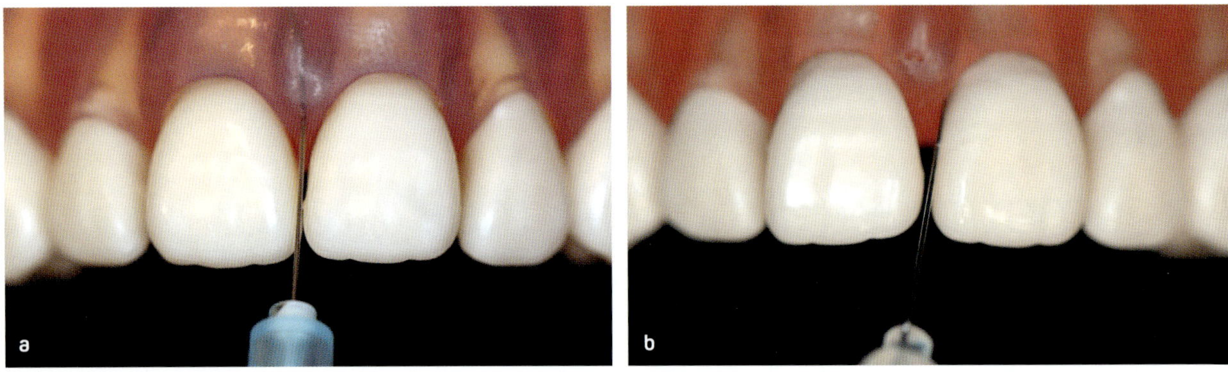

FIG 5-2 Supplementing anesthesia in adjacent gingiva and sulcus. *(a)* Infiltration into the papilla between the central incisors. *(b)* Infiltration in the left central incisor mesiofacial sulcus.

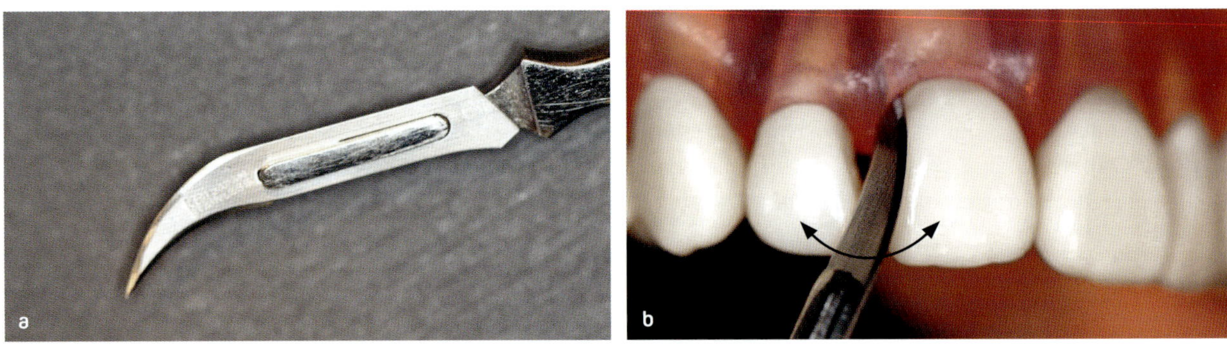

FIG 5-3 *(a)* A 12D scalpel blade. *(b)* The scalpel blade inserted into the distofacial sulcus of the maxillary right central incisor to release the periodontal ligament fibers by applying vertical pressure with a back-and-forth rocking motion.

Release Periodontal Ligament Fibers Without Flap Reflection

Note that some practitioners remove the crown as the first step. They feel that getting the crown out of the way and just dealing with the root(s) is the most efficient and atraumatic method to remove a tooth. For the purposes of this chapter, we will assume the crown will be left in place for these initial procedures.

Using a 12D scalpel blade, enter the sulcus on the mesial, distal, and palatal, but not the facial due to the thin facial bone being vulnerable to resorption and fracture. Apply vertical pressure with a back-and-forth rocking motion (Fig 5-3).

Optional procedure

Use a periotome to excise the fibers as deeply as possible two times around the tooth (Fig 5-4). Use a back-and-forth rocking motion with vertical pressure. However, it may be difficult to get into the periodontal ligament space between the bone and the root surface due to lack of space or ankylosis. If that is the case, proceed to the recommended procedure below.

Recommended procedure

Use a ¼ round high-speed bur to further sever the periodontal ligament fibers (Fig 5-5a).

Use an up-and-down pumping motion circumferentially, avoiding the vulnerable thin facial bone (Fig 5-5b). Extend as far as possible, gently pressuring in

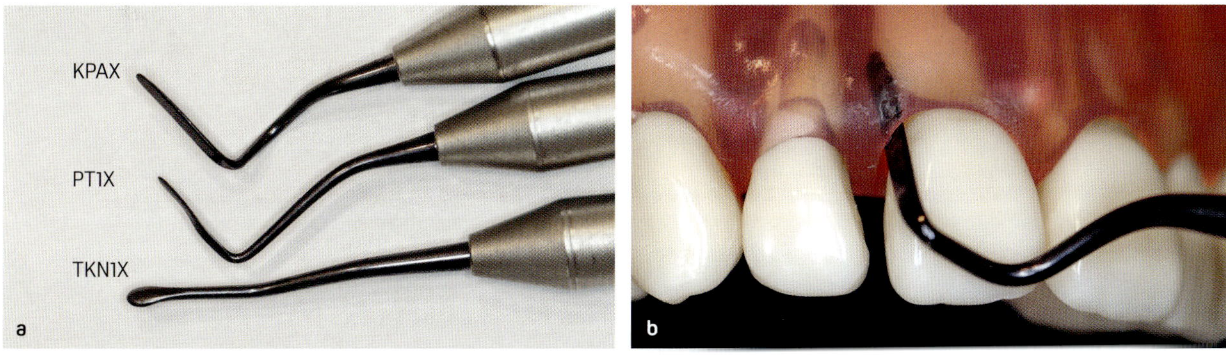

FIG 5-4 *(a)* Hu-Friedy periotomes. *(b)* Hu-Friedy periotome KPAX inserted into the distofacial sulcus of the maxillary right central incisor to excise periodontal ligament fibers. Use vertical pressure and a back-and-forth rocking motion. Avoid the facial due to the thin facial bone.

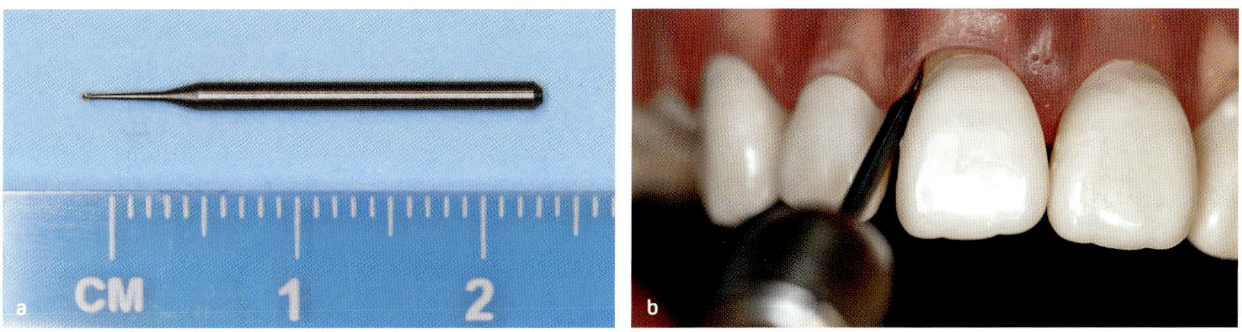

FIG 5-5 *(a)* Surgical-length ¼ round high-speed bur used to separate the root from the bone in the sulcus. *(b)* The bur is inserted in the periodontal ligament space with an up-and-down pumping motion with light pressure against the root, not the bone.

the direction of the tooth root rather than the bone of the socket wall. This opening of the periodontal ligament space releases the tooth from the adjacent bone, making it easier to remove, and creates a space for a thin elevator to enter and pressure the root.

A periotome, scalpel, or ¼ round high-speed bur can be used in any order.

Attempt Tooth Removal Coronally Without Flap Reflection

Introduce a thin elevator (Fig 5-6) at the mesiofacial and distofacial and, using a twisting motion, attempt to move the tooth coronally (Fig 5-7).

At this point, if the tooth cannot be mobilized with a thin elevator or if there is not enough crown present to luxate the tooth but the root is intact, you can use the Easy X-Trac System (A. Titan) or Benex Root Extraction System (Meisinger) (see chapter 12). Both of these systems involve drilling a hole down the middle of the root into the root canal space and inserting a threaded rod. This rod is pulled coronally with a wedging device, removing the root in one piece. To accomplish this, the crown must be cut horizontally approximately 1 mm above the gingival margin, being aware of the gingival margin location to avoid lacerating the gingiva. Since the root is tapered, there is minimal trauma when it is removed in a vertical direction with Easy X-Trac or Benex. In my opinion, this is the most atraumatic method of removing a single-rooted tooth with a tapered root.

However, if there is adequate crown structure present for luxation of any kind, the following may be helpful.

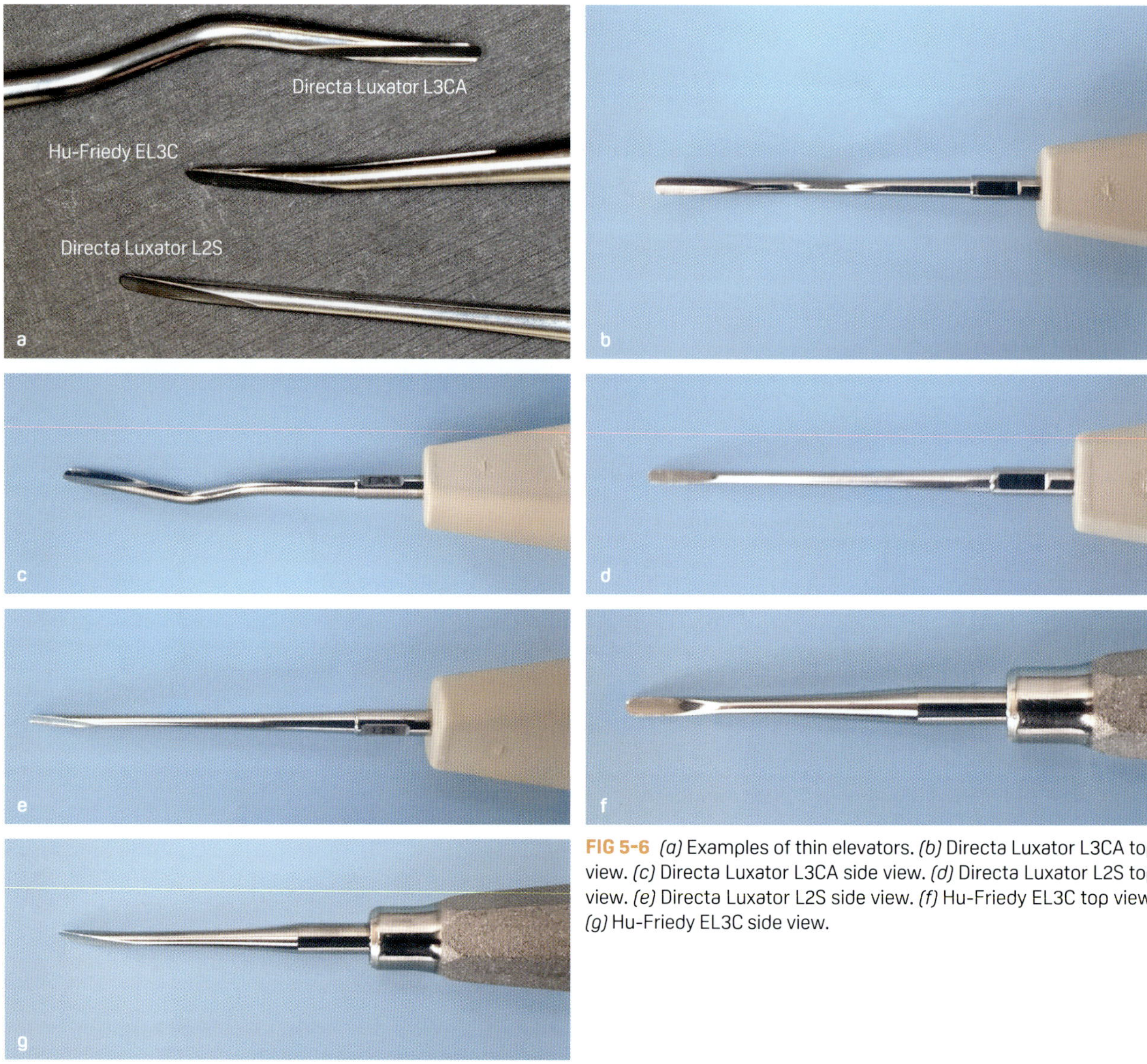

FIG 5-6 *(a)* Examples of thin elevators. *(b)* Directa Luxator L3CA top view. *(c)* Directa Luxator L3CA side view. *(d)* Directa Luxator L2S top view. *(e)* Directa Luxator L2S side view. *(f)* Hu-Friedy EL3C top view. *(g)* Hu-Friedy EL3C side view.

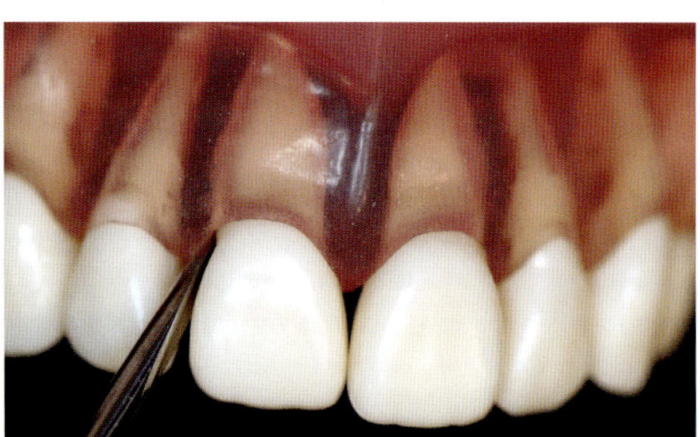

FIG 5-7 Thin elevator (Hu-Friedy EL3C) inserted at the distofacial of the maxillary right central incisor.

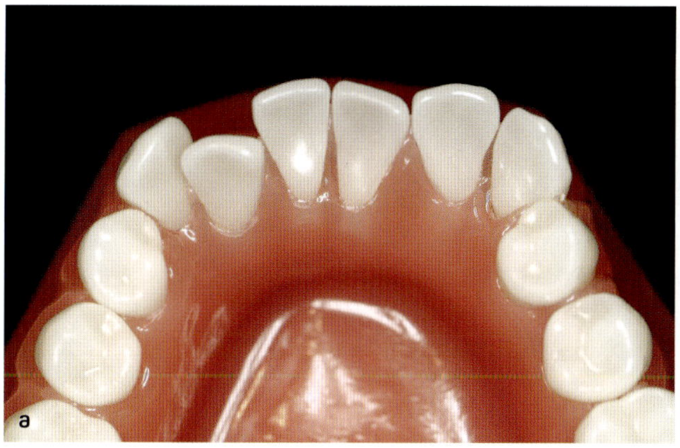

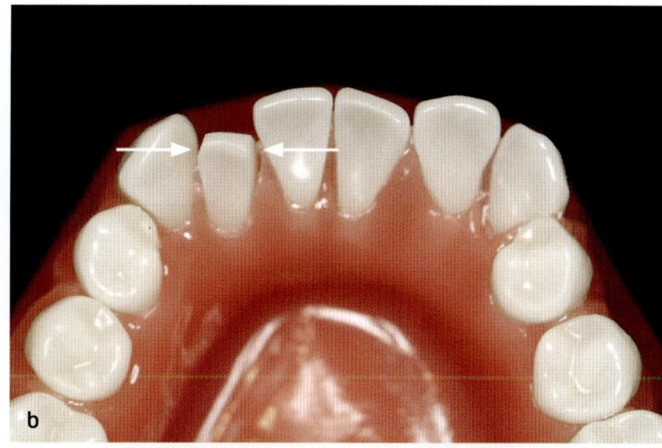

FIG 5-8 *(a)* Mandibular left lateral incisor overlapped with the adjacent canine and central incisor. Rotating the lateral incisor with a forceps will apply pressure to (and may cause increased mobility of) these adjacent teeth. *(b)* The mesial and distal contacts of the lateral incisor have been reduced. *(c)* Now rotation of the lateral incisor with a forceps will be less harmful to adjacent teeth.

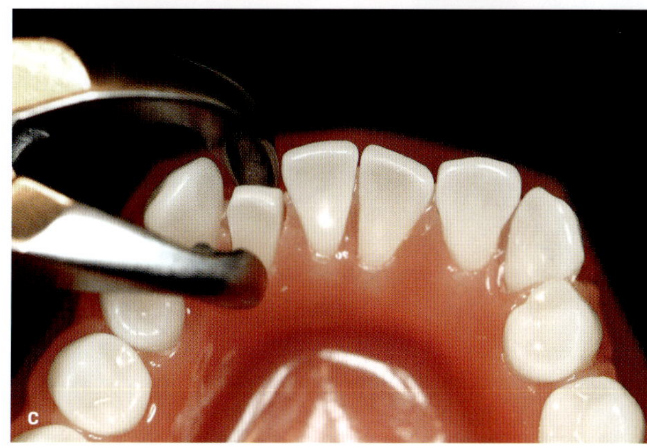

Reduce Interproximal Contacts

We are attempting to remove a tooth as atraumatically as possible, and this pertains not only to the tooth being extracted but also to the adjacent teeth, their restorations, and the rest of the mouth as well. If we were to rotate a tooth with tight or overlapping contacts, we would be pressuring the adjacent contacts and therefore moving the adjacent teeth. (If multiple adjacent teeth are being removed, this concept does not apply; luxation of a tooth with tight or overlapping contacts may actually help loosen adjacent teeth planned for extraction.) Therefore, where teeth are overlapped or crowded, I feel it is important to reduce the interproximal contacts on a single tooth to be removed. Note that if interproximal contacts are present, but luxation does not move or harm adjacent teeth or restorations, then reduction of interproximal contacts is not necessary. If contacts are overlapping on one side only, rotate the tooth in the direction that does not increase contact pressure. Figure 5-8 presents overlapping mandibular incisors as an example.

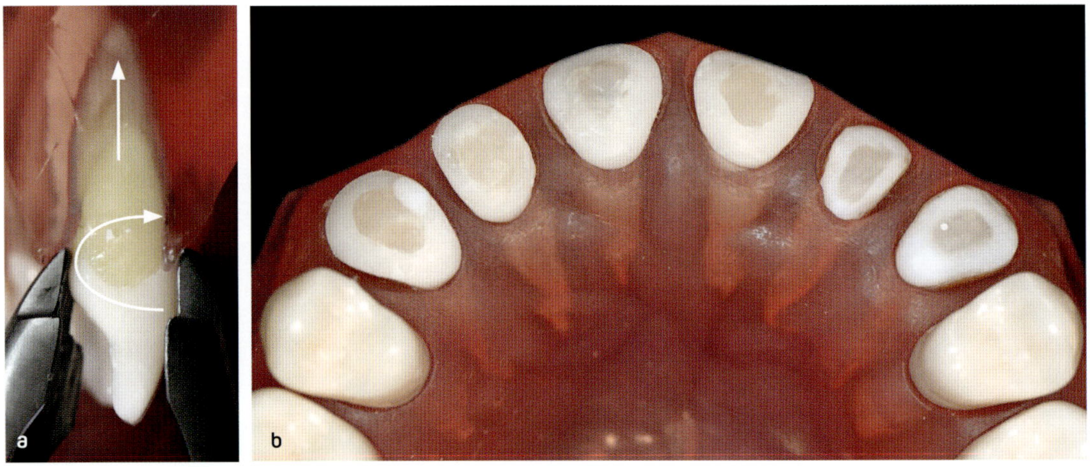

FIG 5-9 *(a)* Forceps applied as apically as possible without damaging bone or soft tissue. First apply vertical pressure, then rotational movement. *(b)* Triangular and oval shape of maxillary anterior tooth roots.

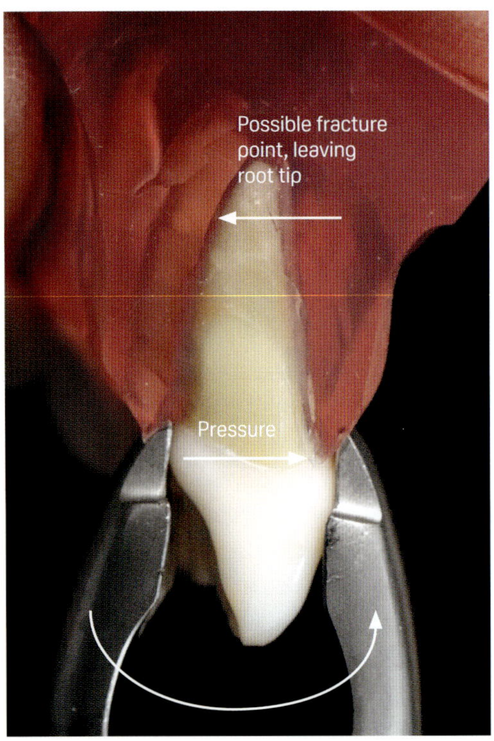

FIG 5-10 Pressure applied coronally toward the facial of the maxillary right central incisor also pressures the palatal surface of the apex. This may result in a fracture of the apex.

Luxate Gently with Forceps

To gently luxate the tooth, place forceps as far apically as possible without engaging bone. Try to engage the root surface apical to any restoration margins. Gently apply pressure apically and hold for 30 seconds. While continuing to apply apical pressure, gently luxate in a twisting motion to test the mobility of the tooth (Fig 5-9a). The reason for applying apical pressure while luxating is that it shifts the axis of rotation in an apical direction, reducing the chance for root fracture. Remember that the roots of anterior maxillary teeth are either triangular or oval in shape; be aware of the root shape and the pressure that might be applied to adjacent roots during rotation (Fig 5-9b).

Rotation of the tooth will expand the socket and may fracture the socket wall. If the bone on the facial or palatal alveolar crest is especially thick, pressure can be applied in that direction. However, realize that when applying pressure coronally in a lateral direction toward the alveolar crest, the apical portion of the tooth will be forced against the opposite socket wall. This pressure can lead to fracture of the apex, leaving a root tip to retrieve (Fig 5-10).

If there is a full-coverage restoration, luxation may or may not remove the crown. If gentle luxation is not successful in removing the tooth, the crown (whether a cemented full-coverage restoration or natural tooth) should be sectioned horizontally about 1 mm coronal to the gingival margin as described in the next section.

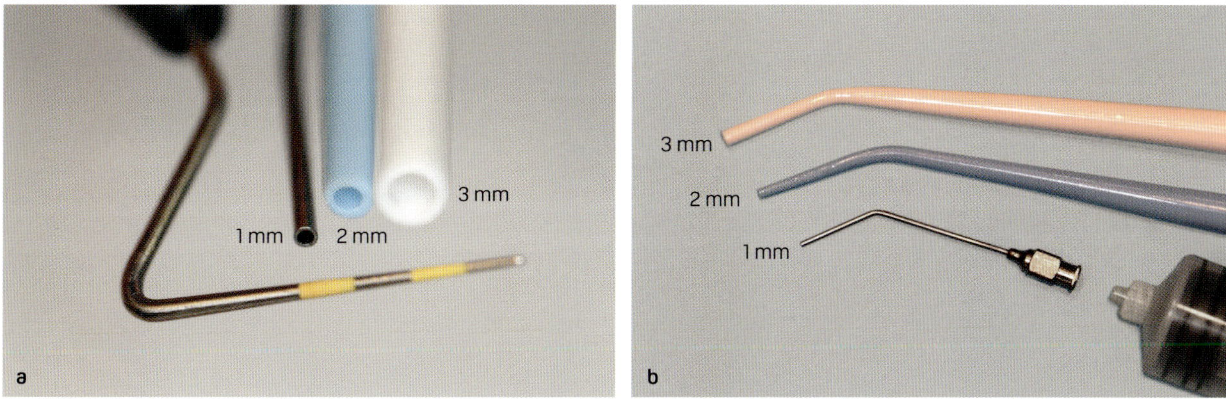

FIG 5-11 *(a and b)* Thin 1-mm irrigation tip and 2- and 3-mm-diameter suction tips used during sectioning of a crown.

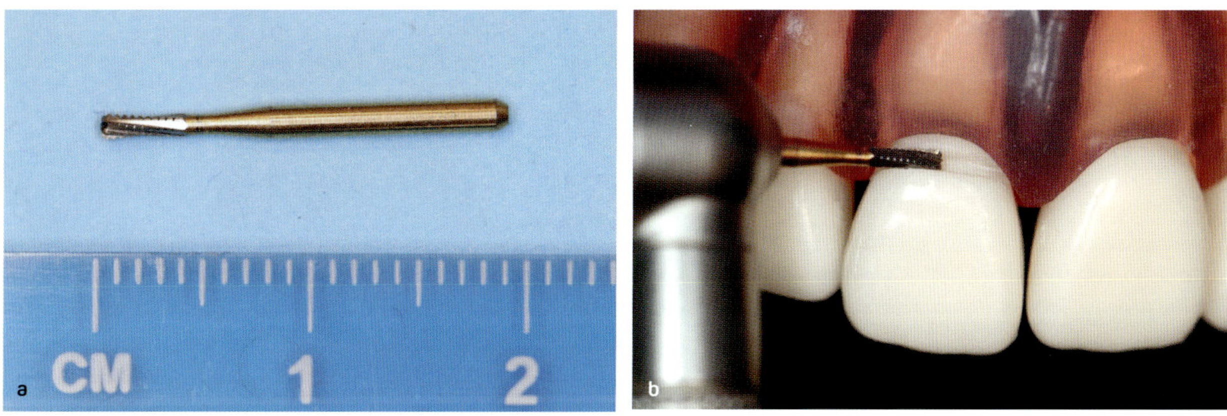

FIG 5-12 *(a)* Great White crosscut fissure bur used to horizontally section the crown. *(b)* Sectioning the maxillary right central incisor 1 mm coronal to the free gingival margin.

Section Crown Horizontally at the Cementoenamel Junction

Some practitioners remove the crown as the first step for every extraction, feeling that it is the most efficient and atraumatic method.

When sectioning a crown or roots, it is important to use plenty of saline irrigation with a thin irrigation tip to remove tooth debris and to use thin suction tips to suction within the drill cuts (Fig 5-11). This allows you to see and feel in these areas. Section the crown 1 mm coronal to the gingival margin using a Great White (SS White) high-speed crosscut fissure bur (Fig 5-12). It is important to be aware of the gingival margin location to avoid lacerating the gingiva.

Obviously, it's much easier to section through tooth structure or a composite restoration as compared to a metal restoration. Regardless of the material, section two-thirds of the way through the crown, and then, using an elevator, gently pry off the crown. Using a football-shaped diamond bur, smooth the remaining tooth structure to create a fairly flat surface approximately 1 mm coronal to the gingival margin (Fig 5-13).

Removing the crown allows you to see the remaining root structure anatomy and determine the best location to section vertically. Vertical fractures may be evident also. A dye such as To Dye For (Roydent) may be used to help visualize possible fractures.

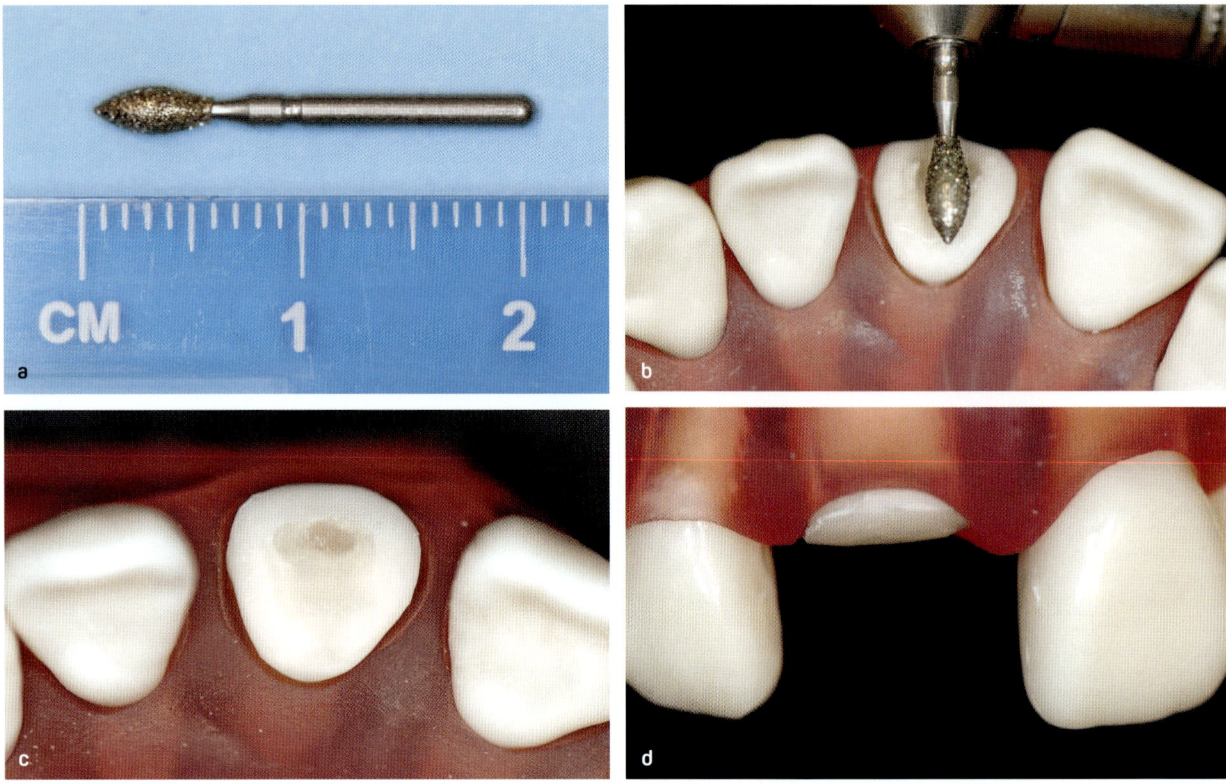

FIG 5-13 *(a and b)* Football diamond bur used to smooth the remaining root to a level 1 mm above the gingival margin after sectioning off the crown. *(c and d)* Occlusal and facial views of the maxillary right central incisor sectioned horizontally 1 mm above the gingival margin.

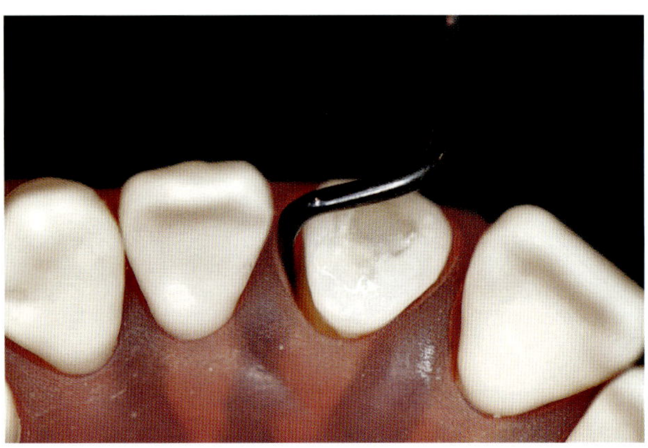

FIG 5-14 Using a periotome to apply vertical pressure and a back-and-forth rocking motion in the sulcus.

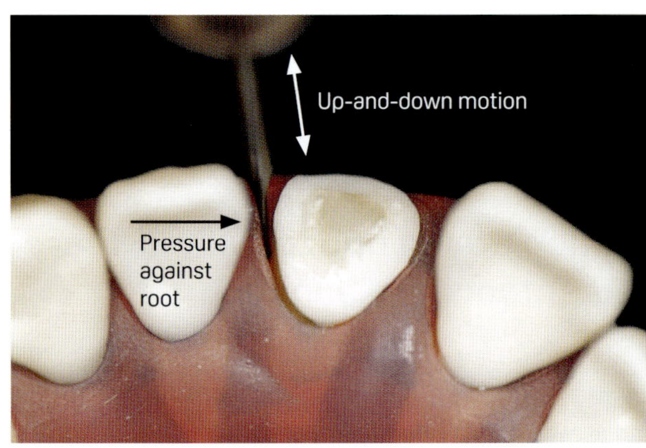

FIG 5-15 A ¼ round high-speed bur used with a gentle up-and-down motion in the sulcus, exerting pressure toward the root, not the bone of the socket wall.

Optional procedure

Release the periodontal ligament fibers again using a narrow periotome (see Fig 5-4a). Enter the sulcus on the palatal, mesial, and distal, applying vertical pressure and a back-and-forth rocking motion to excise the periodontal ligament fibers further apically (Fig 5-14).

Recommended procedure

Instead of a periotome, you can use a surgical-length ¼ round high-speed bur in an up-and-down motion to further sever the periodontal ligament fibers (Fig 5-15). Attempt to cut more in the direction of the root rather than the bone of the socket wall. Excising periodontal ligament fibers like this detaches the root from the bone, allowing for easier extraction. Avoid the facial aspect because bone in this area is thin.

Use Thin Elevator to Attempt Root Removal Coronally Without Flap Reflection

Introducing a thin elevator (see Fig 5-6a) at the mesiofacial and distofacial, use a twisting motion to attempt to move the root coronally (Fig 5-16). If the root moves but not coronally, release the periodontal ligament fibers again with the periotome or ¼ round bur, then try the elevators again at the mesiofacial and distofacial. If you are not able to remove the root at this point, the next step is to insert the beaks of an incisor forceps as apically as possible and attempt luxation and slight rotation one more time (Fig 5-17).

If this is not successful, the next step is to vertically section the root.

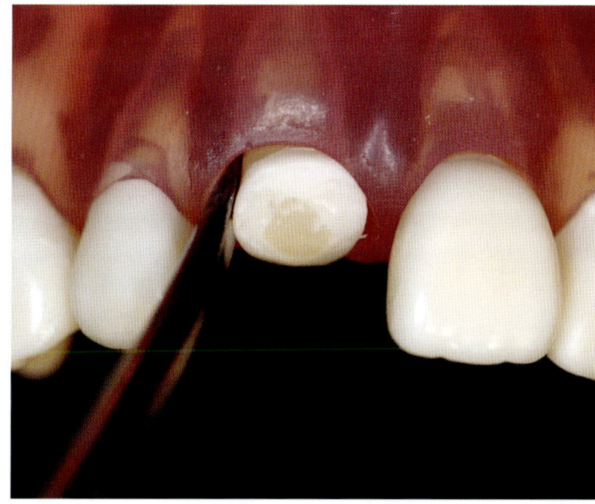

FIG 5-16 A thin Hu-Friedy EL3C elevator is used to gently luxate the root of the maxillary right central incisor with a twisting motion, attempting to elevate it out of the socket.

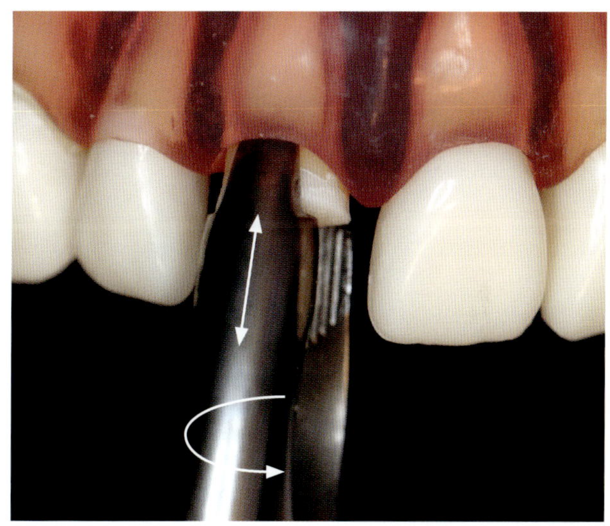

FIG 5-17 Using an incisor forceps to mobilize the maxillary right central incisor root.

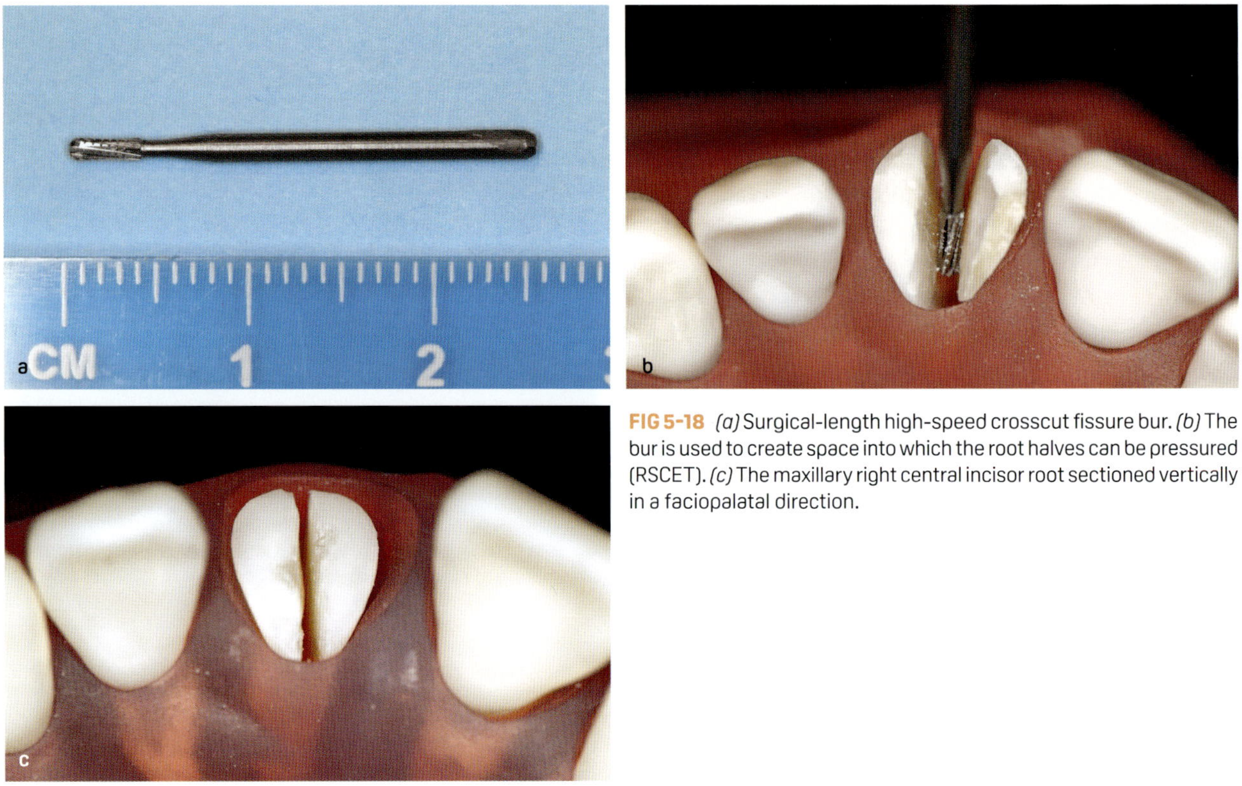

FIG 5-18 *(a)* Surgical-length high-speed crosscut fissure bur. *(b)* The bur is used to create space into which the root halves can be pressured (RSCET). *(c)* The maxillary right central incisor root sectioned vertically in a faciopalatal direction.

Section Roots Vertically

This technique is termed the *root space creation extraction technique (RSCET)*. The concept involves using a surgical-length high-speed crosscut fissure bur (Fig 5-18a) to remove tooth structure and creating a space into which the root can be pressured, away from the sulcus and socket wall. In this way, a tooth can be removed without removing supporting bone. Single-rooted teeth usually are sectioned in a faciopalatal direction so that mobilization of the root fragments does not stress the facial bone, but care must be taken to avoid scoring the facial bone (Figs 5-18b and 5-18c). It is important that you have thin sterile saline irrigation and suction tips that reach the apices of the roots you are sectioning, allowing you to irrigate and suction the drill cuts and removing tooth debris for visualization.

If the root is not sectioned entirely through the apex, pressuring the root into the space may result in a horizontal fracture at the depth of the cut (Fig 5-19a). Therefore, if the surgical-length high-speed crosscut fissure bur does not reach the apex, use a straight handpiece round bur #4 or #6 to complete cutting through the apex. This requires opening up the cut wider at the coronal aspect to allow room for the shank of the straight handpiece bur (Figs 5-19b and 5-19c). When you feel the bur "drop" into the softer bone, you know you have sectioned through the apex (Fig 5-19d). Cut toward the palatal and facial slightly to make sure the cut is through the root structure.

Once you have confirmed the root has been completely divided through the apex, proceed as follows.

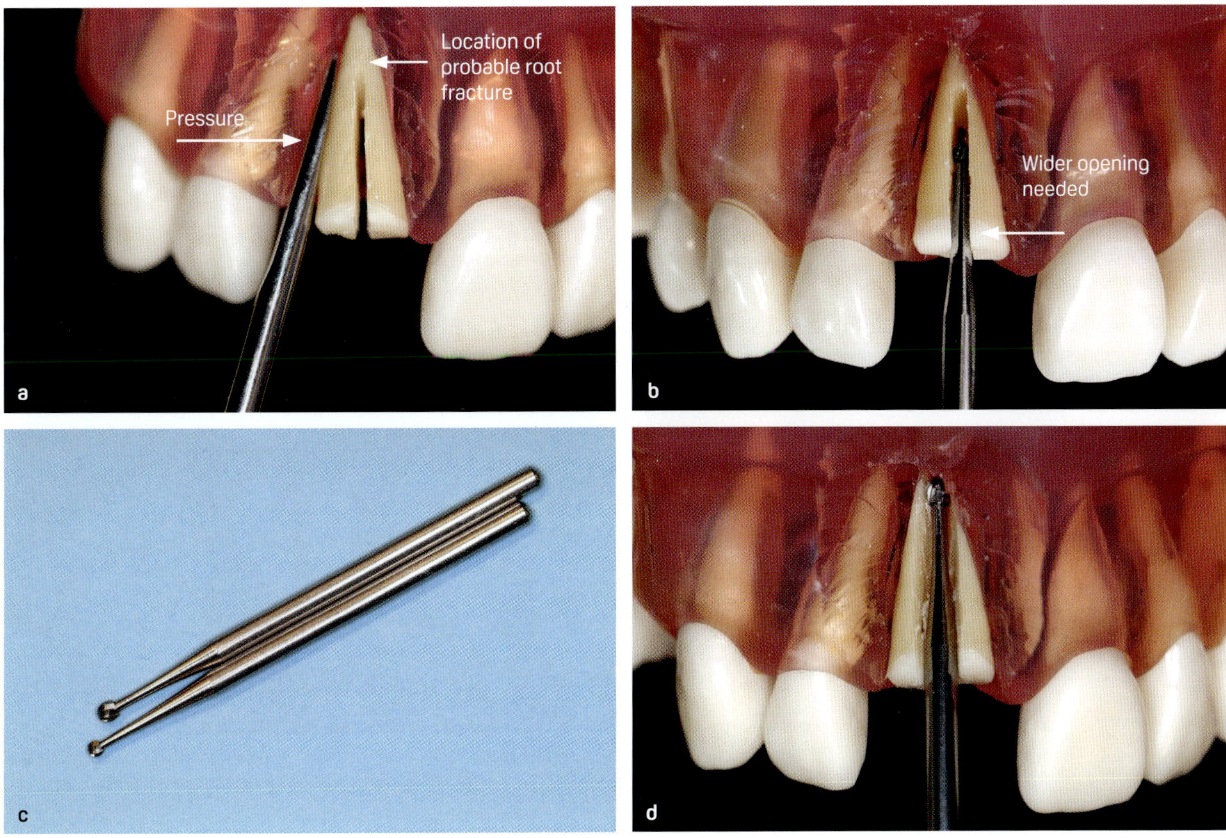

FIG 5-19 *(a)* Thin elevator (Directa L2S) at the distal of the maxillary right central incisor, pressuring the incompletely sectioned root. There is a risk of fracturing the root at the depth of the cut, leaving the apex attached to the remaining root (gingiva removed for visualization purposes). *(b)* Root not sectioned entirely through apex. A wider opening is needed to allow room for the shank of the straight handpiece bur. *(c)* Straight handpiece burs #6 *(top)* and #4 *(bottom)*; the smaller bur (#4) is used for smaller roots, and #6 is used for larger roots. *(d)* Straight handpiece bur #6 sectioning completely past the apex into bone.

Elevate Gently Between Sectioned Root Pieces

Pressure sectioned roots laterally using a twisting motion with the thin elevator Directa L2S or Hu-Friedy EL3C (Fig 5-20). Be aware that you are also pressuring the bone laterally, so if it looks like there is a weak area of bone, avoid pressuring that area.

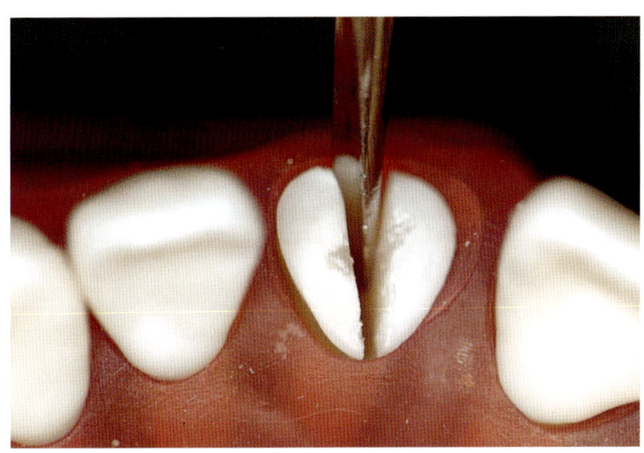

FIG 5-20 Thin elevator used with a gentle twisting motion to pressure root sections laterally.

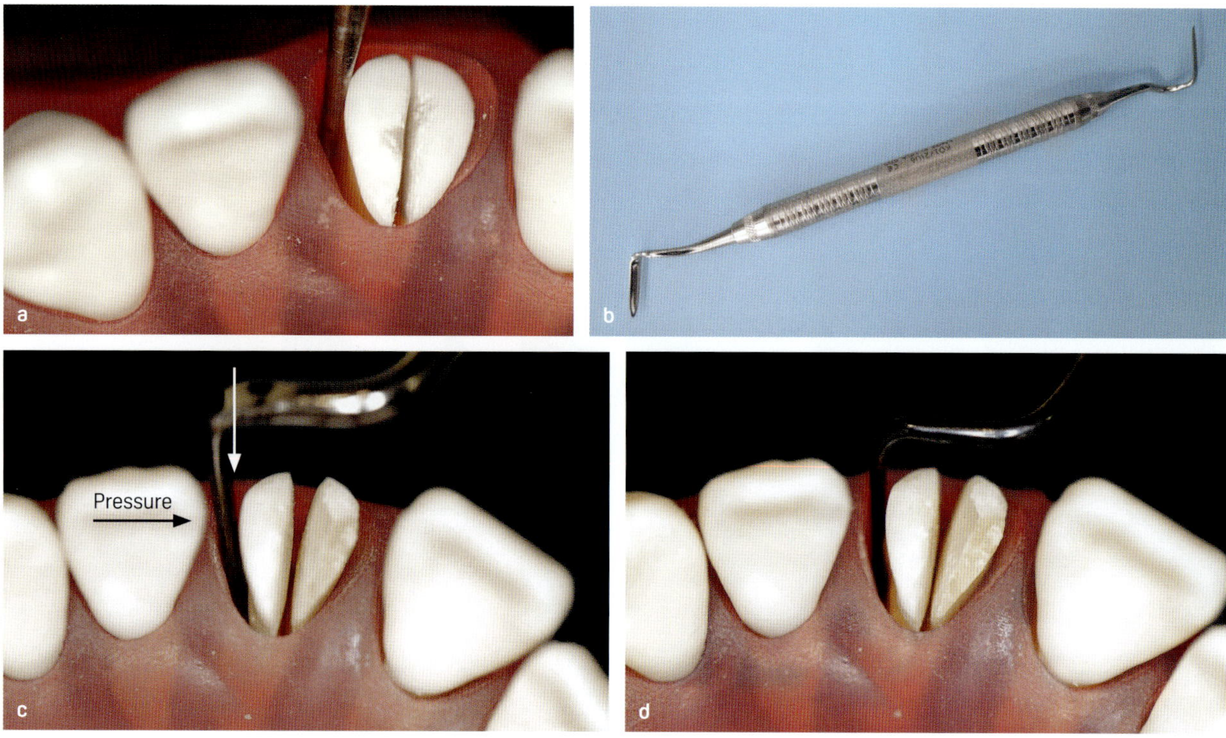

FIG 5-21 Various instruments used with vertical pressure and a back-and-forth rocking motion to pressure the root halves inward into the space created by sectioning of the root (RSCET). *(a)* Thin Directa L2S elevator. *(b and c)* Hu-Friedy Orban knife KO1/2IU. *(d)* Periotome.

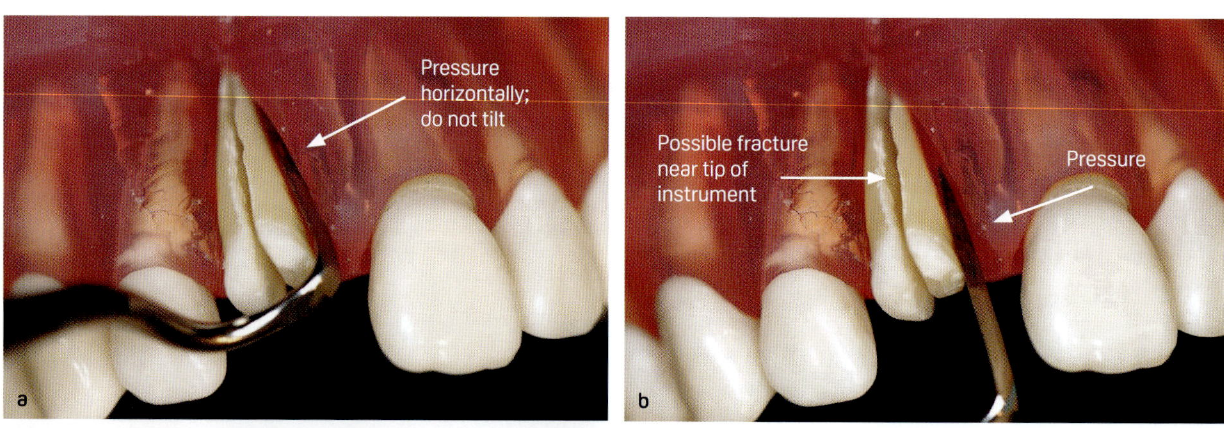

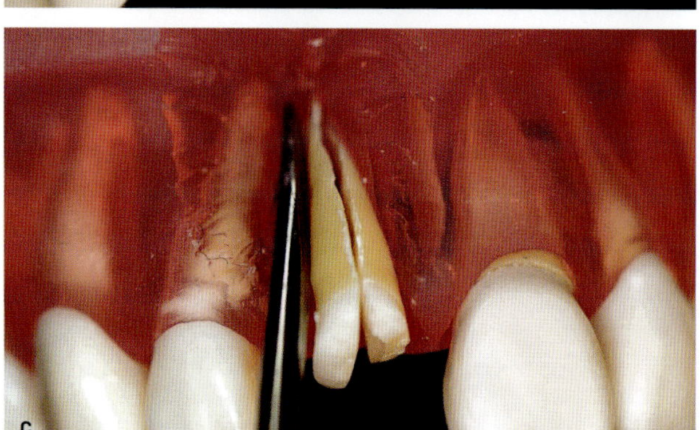

FIG 5-22 *(a)* Placement of the Orban knife as far apically as possible in the periodontal ligament space to pressure, rather than tilt, the root. *(b)* If the Orban knife is positioned only halfway down the root surface, there is a greater chance the root will fracture as it is pressured into the space created by sectioning the root. Pressure on the coronal half of the sectioned root stresses the mid-root area, leading to possible fracture, even if it is fully sectioned through the apex. *(c)* Thin elevator inserted fully in the periodontal ligament space, reaching the apex.

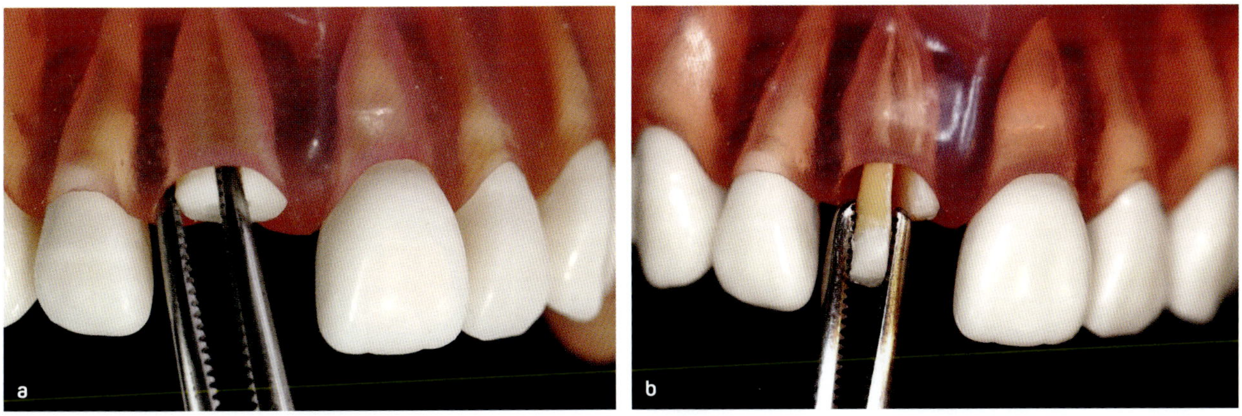

FIG 5-23 *(a)* Hemostat locked onto a mobile root segment. *(b)* A gentle back-and-forth motion with constant pulling pressure is used to remove the root segment from the socket.

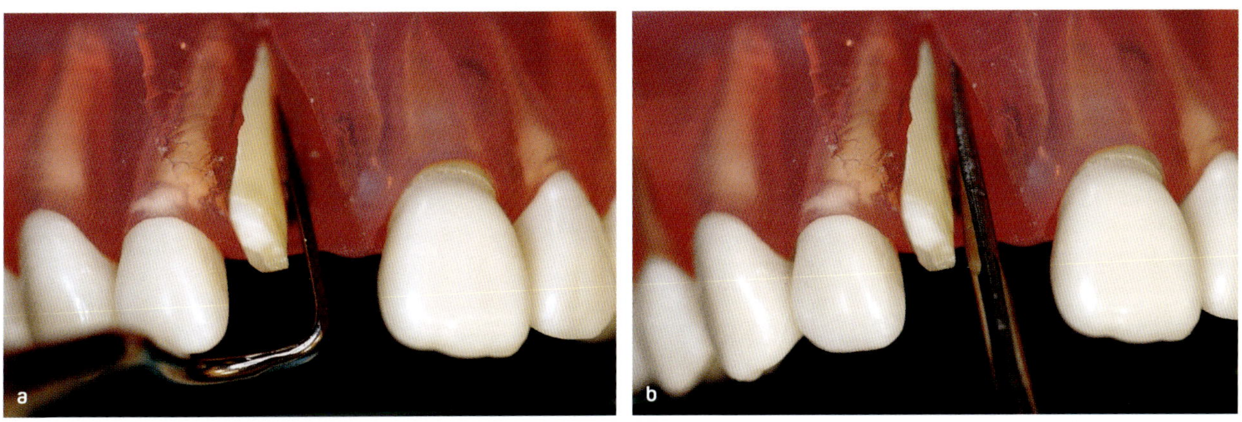

FIG 5-24 *(a)* Using an Orban knife to pressure the remaining root section into the space created when the initial half of the root was removed (RSCET). *(b)* Same procedure performed using a thin elevator. Once this remaining root section has been mobilized into the space, it can be removed with a hemostat or tweezers.

Enter Sulcus Laterally and Pressure Roots into Sectioned Space

Using a Hu-Friedy Orban knife KO1/2IU, periotome, or thin elevator, enter the sulcus on the mesial and distal surfaces of the roots and attempt to force the root halves into the space created by sectioning the root (Fig 5-21). It is important to make sure the instrument is seated as far as possible into the sulcus so the root is pressured rather than tilted, which may cause the root tip to fracture (Fig 5-22).

Be aware that you are pressuring against the adjacent bone, so do this in a gentle manner, paying attention to the integrity of the adjacent bone. As before, use thin irrigation and suction tips that reach the apex of the roots you are sectioning to irrigate and suction drill cuts. You may find that reentering the sectioned area and cutting between the root sections again may be required. If this does not mobilize the root fragments, it may be necessary to section the root fragments themselves (see next section).

Once root segments are mobilized, individual pieces can be removed with a hemostat. Lock a hemostat onto a mobile root segment as far apically as possible and use a gentle back-and-forth motion with constant pulling pressure to remove the root segment from the socket (Fig 5-23). This technique is helpful in many instances in which a tooth fragment has been mobilized and needs to be removed.

After one root section is removed, pressure the remaining root section into the space created by removal of the first (RSCET; Fig 5-24). Then remove this second root half.

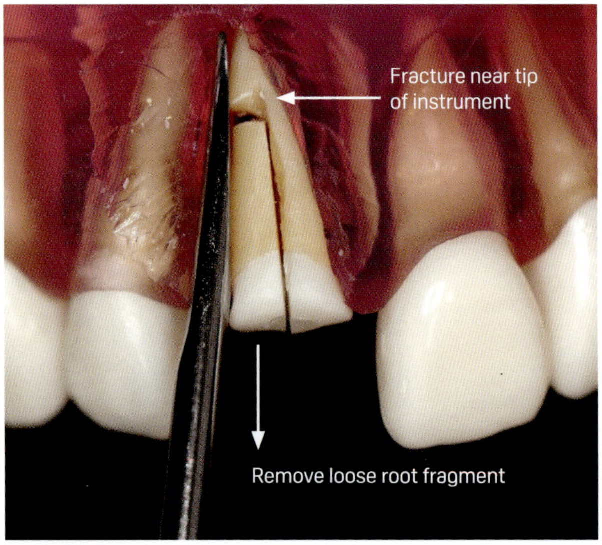

FIG 5-25 If horizontal fracture occurs, the first step is to remove the loose root fragment.

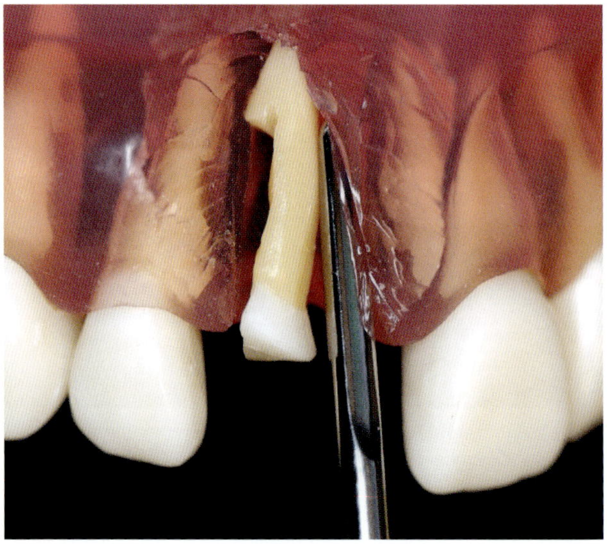

FIG 5-26 Pressuring the remaining root, with apex attached, into the space created by removing the root fragment (RSCET).

Section Roots Again; Pressure into Space Created

If root halves cannot be mobilized and removed, consider vertically sectioning one and possibly both root halves so they are in quarters, being careful to avoid the mesial and distal socket walls. This is more applicable to larger roots, but smaller roots may require this step, at which time you are actually drilling out most of the root. Again, it is necessary to drill through the apex; feeling the bur drop into softer bone is an indication that you are past the apex. Then, pressure those root quarters into the space created (RSCET) and remove them.

Once root removal is complete, proceed to socket debridement (see chapter 11).

Complications

If the root is not sectioned entirely through the apex or if the apex fractures, atraumatic removal is difficult. The following steps will help reduce the severity of such complications.

As mentioned earlier, if the root is not sectioned entirely through the apex, pressuring the root into the space may result in a horizontal fracture at the depth of the cut (see Fig 5-19a). If horizontal fracture occurs, remove the loose root fragment (Fig 5-25). The choice is then to attempt to pressure the remaining root, with the apex attached, into the space created by removing the root fragment or to section through the apex.

If the remaining root is pressured into the space created by removing the root fragment (RSCET; Fig 5-26), the risk is another horizontal root fracture, leaving the entire apex. This approach is more successful in softer maxillary bone. Attempting this in the denser mandibular bone will result in fractures more frequently. The other option is to section through the apex (Fig 5-27).

A fractured apex is a complication we will all experience. Sectioning entirely through the apex is necessary to help prevent these complications.

Once root removal is complete, proceed to socket debridement (see chapter 11).

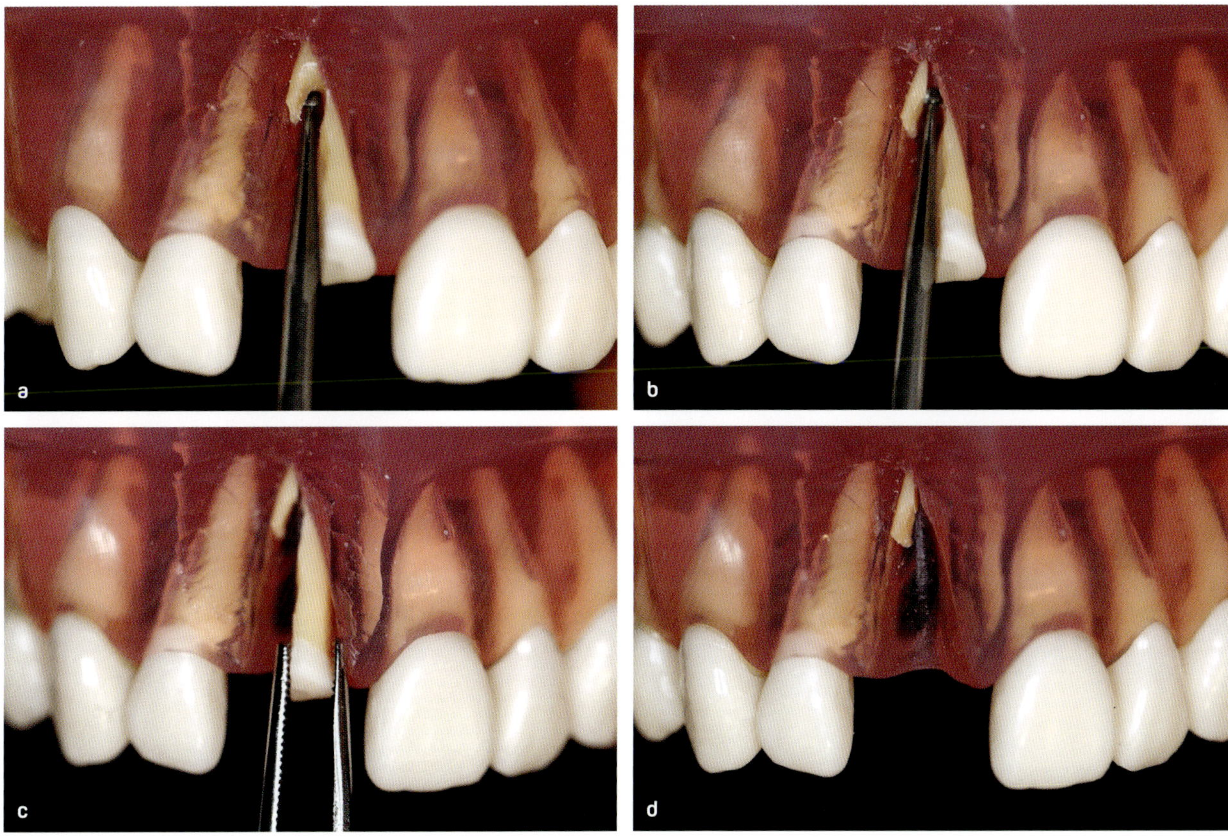

FIG 5-27 *(a and b)* If horizontal fracture occurs, remove the loose root fragment and use a straight handpiece bur #4 or #6 to completely section through the apex. *(c)* Once you are through the apex, remove the long root fragment. *(d)* Half apex remaining. This can be mobilized using a thin elevator and then removed.

6

Atraumatic Extractions in the Anterior Mandible: Watch Out for Thin Bone

The following atraumatic extraction techniques apply to mandibular canines and incisors with minimal to no mobility and good bone support. Obviously, teeth with Class II or III mobility can usually be removed atraumatically if there is adequate crown structure to grasp with a forceps. Also, it may not be necessary to use all of the following techniques to atraumatically remove a tooth. Some of the steps may be deemed nonproductive or not applicable to the clinical situation and therefore can be skipped at the discretion of the operating dentist.

The mandibular right central incisor is the demonstration example in this chapter; however, these principles apply to all mandibular canines and incisors since they have similarly shaped roots.

Verify Profound Anesthesia

Probe the sulcus with a periodontal probe and stimulate the adjacent gingiva, especially on the lingual, to confirm you have profound anesthesia (Fig 6-1). If anesthesia is inadequate, administer either another nerve block or infiltration into the sulcus and adjacent gingiva circumferentially (Fig 6-2). For quickest onset, use 4% articaine with 1:100,000 epinephrine. For hemostasis, 2% lidocaine 1:100,000 epinephrine is helpful.

A bite block can be used to stabilize the mandible; this also helps patients hold their mouth open during the procedure, reducing muscle fatigue.

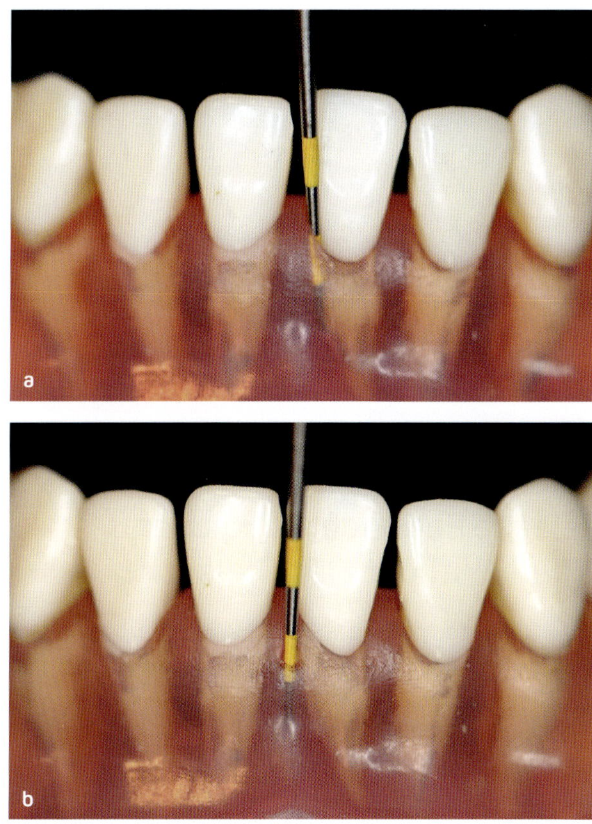

FIG 6-1 Verifying adequate anesthesia. *(a)* Probing the mesiofacial sulcus of the mandibular left central incisor. *(b)* Probing the gingiva.

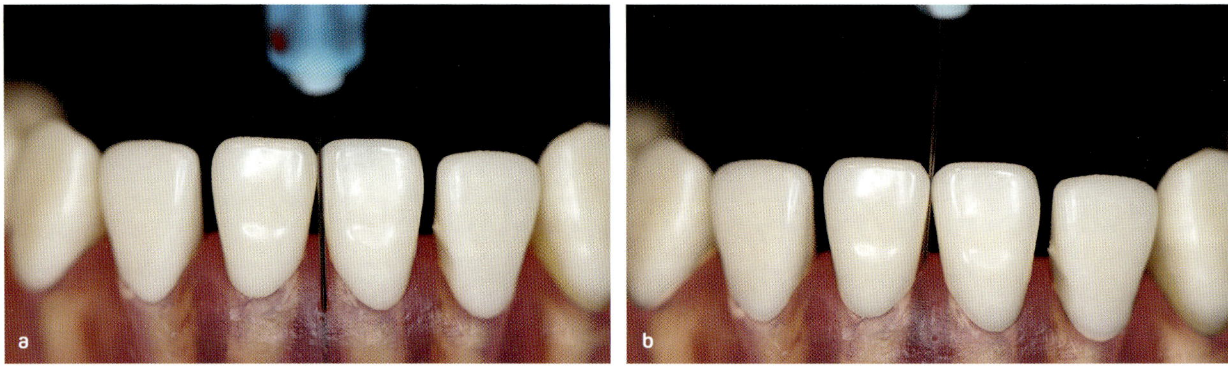

FIG 6-2 Supplementing anesthesia in adjacent gingiva and sulcus. *(a)* Infiltration into the papilla between the central incisors. *(b)* Infiltration into the mesial sulcus of the mandibular right central incisor.

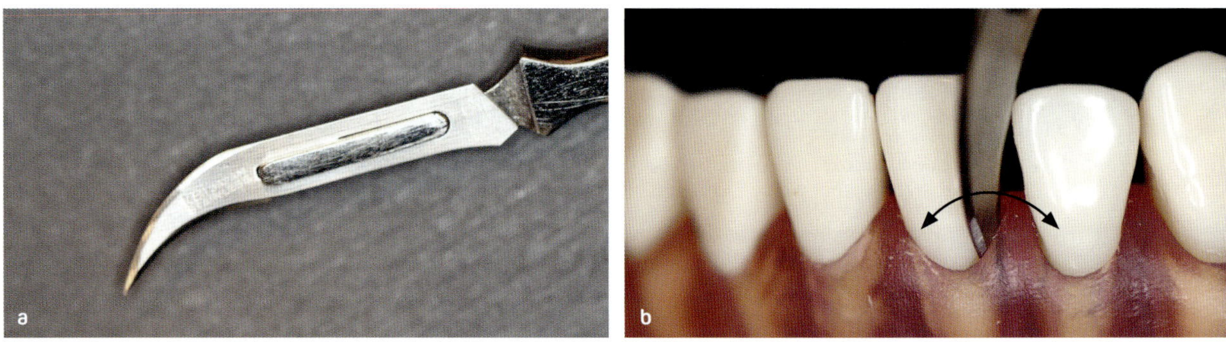

FIG 6-3 *(a)* A 12D scalpel blade. *(b)* The scalpel blade inserted into the distofacial sulcus of the mandibular left central incisor to release the periodontal ligament fibers by applying vertical pressure with a back-and-forth rocking motion.

Release Periodontal Ligament Fibers Without Flap Reflection

Note that some practitioners remove the crown as the first step. They feel that getting the crown out of the way and just dealing with the root(s) is the most efficient and atraumatic method to remove a tooth. For the purposes of this chapter, we will assume the crown will be left in place for these initial procedures.

Using a 12D scalpel blade, enter the sulcus on the mesial, distal, and lingual, but not the facial due to the thin facial bone being vulnerable to resorption and fracture. Apply vertical pressure with a back-and-forth rocking motion (Fig 6-3).

Optional procedure

Use a periotome to excise the fibers as deeply as possible two times around the tooth (Fig 6-4). Use a back-and-forth rocking motion with vertical pressure. However, it may be difficult to get into the periodontal ligament space due to lack of space or ankylosis. If that is the case, proceed to the recommended procedure below.

Recommended procedure

Use a ¼ round high-speed bur to further sever the periodontal ligament fibers (Fig 6-5a). Use an up-and-down pumping motion in the periodontal ligament space at the mesial, distal, and lingual, but avoid the facial since the thin facial bone is vulnerable to resorption and fracture (Fig 6-5b). Extend as far apically as possible, gently pressuring in the direction of the tooth root rather than the bone of the socket wall. This opening of the periodontal ligament space releases the tooth from the adjacent bone, making it easier to remove, and creates a space for a thin elevator to enter and pressure the root.

A periotome, scalpel, or ¼ round high-speed bur can be used in any order.

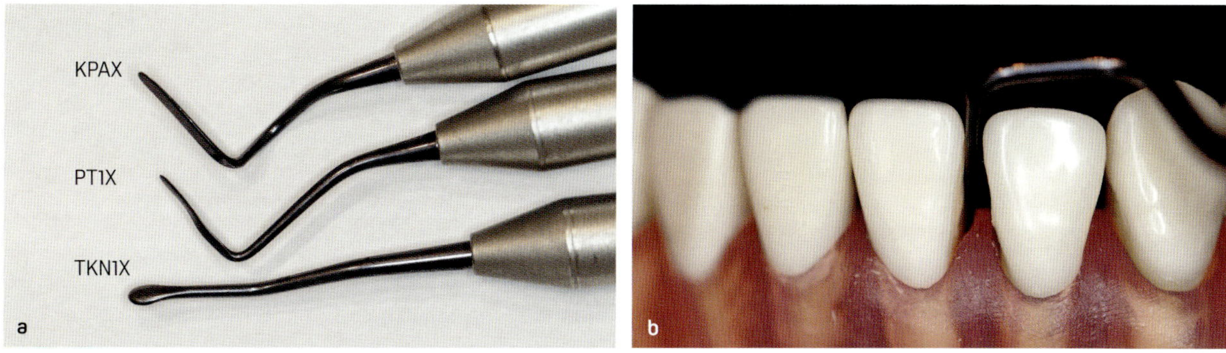

FIG 6-4 *(a)* Hu-Friedy periotomes. *(b)* Periotome inserted into the distal sulcus of the mandibular left central incisor to excise the periodontal ligament fibers. Use vertical pressure and a back-and-forth rocking motion. Avoid the thin facial bone.

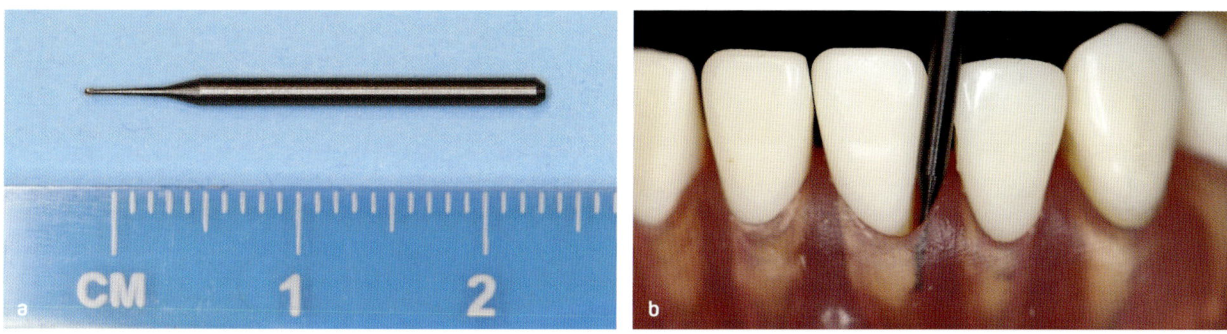

FIG 6-5 *(a)* Surgical-length ¼ round high-speed bur used to separate the root from the bone in the sulcus. *(b)* The bur is inserted in the sulcus with an up-and-down pumping motion with light pressure against the root, not the bone.

Attempt Tooth Removal Coronally Without Flap Reflection

Introduce a thin elevator (Fig 6-6) at the mesiobuccal and distobuccal and, using a twisting motion, attempt to move the tooth coronally (Fig 6-7).

At this point, if the tooth cannot be mobilized with a thin elevator or if there is not enough crown present to luxate the tooth but the root is intact, you can use the Easy X-Trac System (A. Titan) or Benex Root Extraction System (Meisinger) (see chapter 12). However, keep in mind that the canines are the only mandibular anterior teeth that are generally wide enough to be removed with either one of these techniques; the mandibular incisors (nos. 23–26) are generally too thin mesiodistally to be removed with Easy X-Trac or Benex. Both of these systems involve drilling a hole down the middle of the root canal space and inserting a threaded rod. This rod is pulled coronally with a wedging device, removing the root in one piece. To accomplish this, the crown must be cut horizontally approximately 1 mm above the gingival margin, being aware of the gingival margin location to avoid lacerating the gingiva. Since the root is tapered, there is minimal trauma when it is removed in a vertical direction with the Easy X-Trac or Benex. In my opinion, this is the most atraumatic method of removing a single-rooted tooth with a tapered root.

However, if there is adequate crown structure present for luxation of any kind, the following may be helpful.

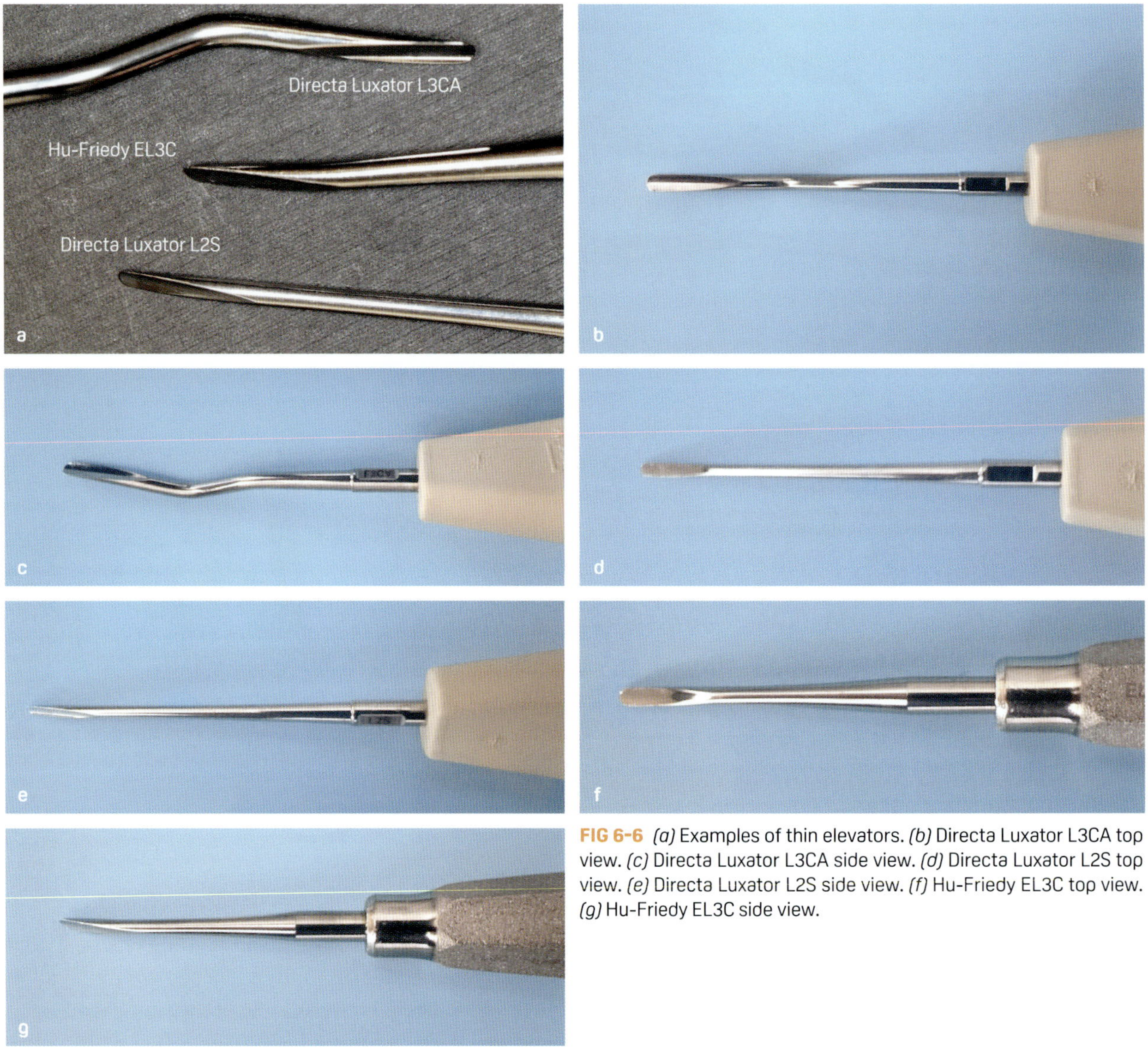

FIG 6-6 *(a)* Examples of thin elevators. *(b)* Directa Luxator L3CA top view. *(c)* Directa Luxator L3CA side view. *(d)* Directa Luxator L2S top view. *(e)* Directa Luxator L2S side view. *(f)* Hu-Friedy EL3C top view. *(g)* Hu-Friedy EL3C side view.

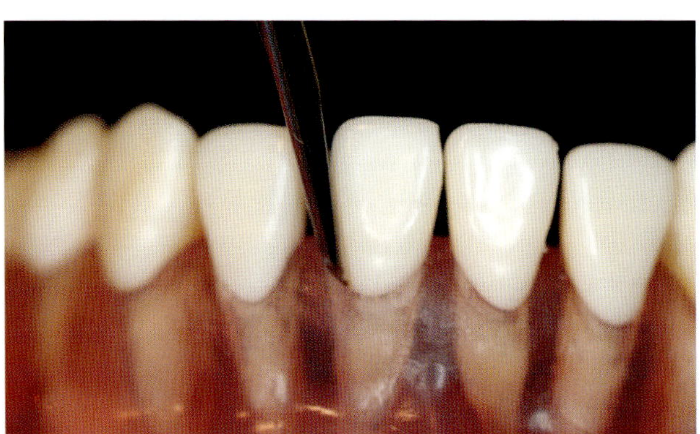

FIG 6-7 Thin elevator (Hu-Friedy EL3C) inserted at the distofacial of the mandibular right central incisor.

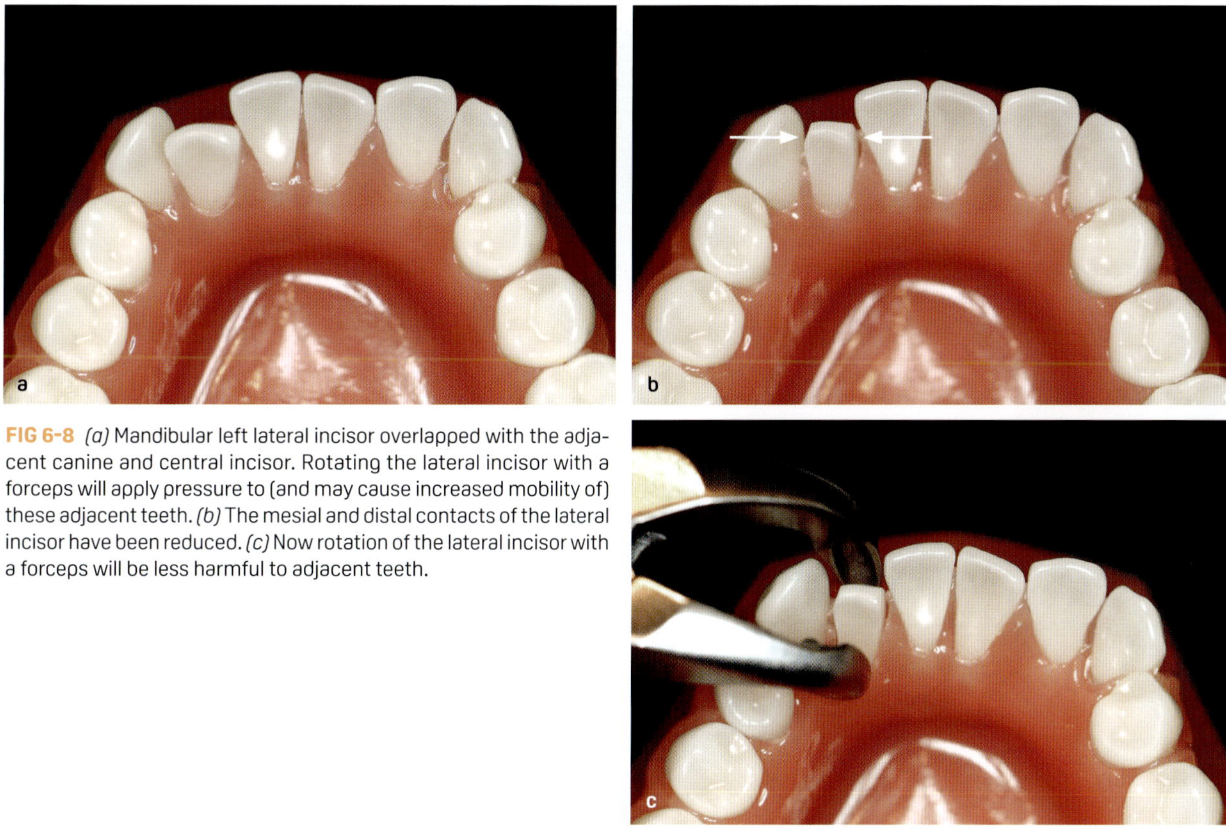

FIG 6-8 *(a)* Mandibular left lateral incisor overlapped with the adjacent canine and central incisor. Rotating the lateral incisor with a forceps will apply pressure to (and may cause increased mobility of) these adjacent teeth. *(b)* The mesial and distal contacts of the lateral incisor have been reduced. *(c)* Now rotation of the lateral incisor with a forceps will be less harmful to adjacent teeth.

Reduce Interproximal Contacts

We are attempting to remove a tooth as atraumatically as possible, and this pertains not only to the tooth being extracted but also to the adjacent teeth, their restorations, and the rest of the mouth as well. If we were to rotate a tooth with tight or overlapping contacts, we would be pressuring the adjacent contacts and therefore moving the adjacent teeth. (If multiple adjacent teeth are being removed, this concept does not apply; luxation of a tooth with tight or overlapping contacts may actually help loosen adjacent teeth planned for extraction.) Therefore, where teeth are overlapped or crowded, I feel it is important to reduce the interproximal contacts on a single tooth to be removed. Note that if interproximal contacts are present, but luxation does not move or harm adjacent teeth or restorations, then reduction of interproximal contacts is not necessary. If contacts are overlapping on one side only, rotate the tooth in the direction that does not increase contact pressure. Figure 6-8 presents overlapping mandibular incisors as an example.

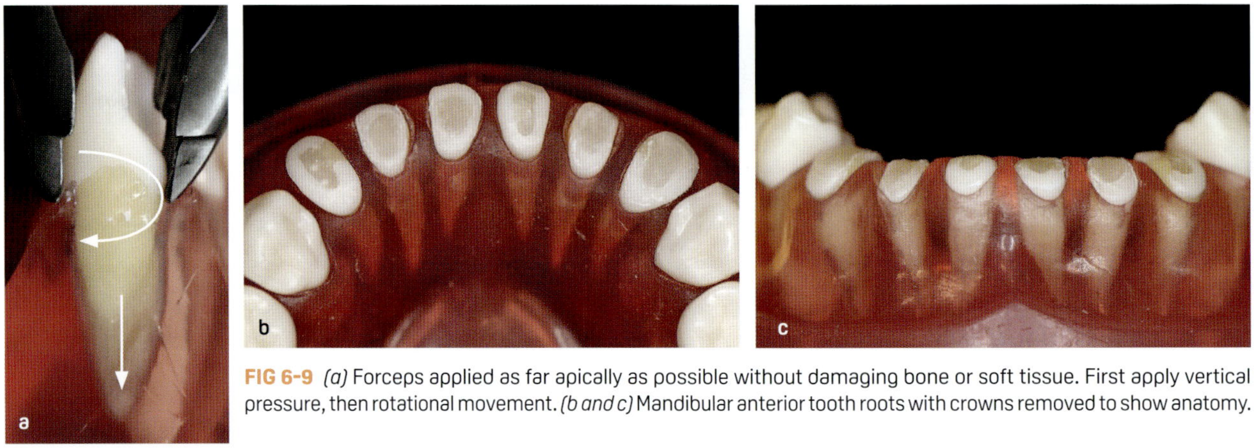

FIG 6-9 *(a)* Forceps applied as far apically as possible without damaging bone or soft tissue. First apply vertical pressure, then rotational movement. *(b and c)* Mandibular anterior tooth roots with crowns removed to show anatomy.

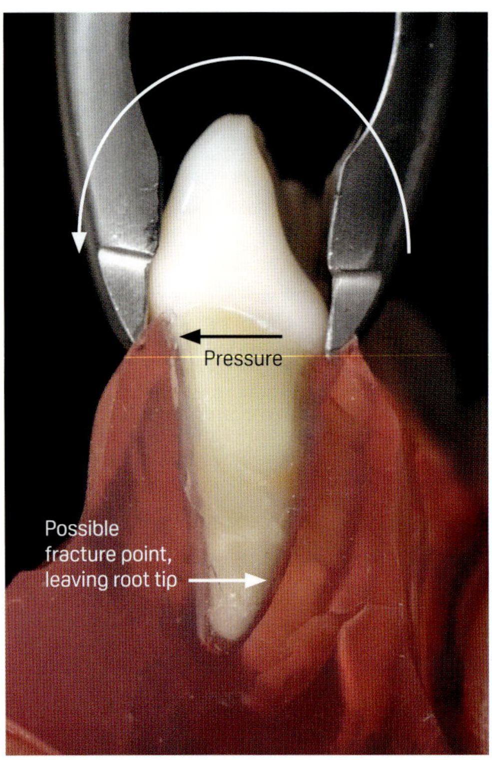

FIG 6-10 Pressure applied coronally toward the facial of the mandibular right central incisor also pressures the lingual surface of the apex. This may result in a fracture of the apex.

Luxate Gently with Forceps

To gently luxate the tooth, place forceps as far apically as possible without engaging bone. Try to engage the root surface apical to any restoration margins. Gently apply pressure apically and hold for 30 seconds. While continuing to apply apical pressure, gently luxate in a twisting motion to test the mobility of the tooth (Fig 6-9a). The reason for applying apical pressure while luxating is that it shifts the axis of rotation in an apical direction, reducing the chance for root fracture. Remember that the roots of the mandibular anterior teeth are oval in shape and much wider faciolingually than mesiodistally (Figs 6-9b and 6-9c). Rotating them will expand the socket and may fracture the socket wall. Generally, bone on the facial and lingual of the mandibular anterior teeth is especially thin. This is most evident on the lingual of the mandibular central incisors, where the bone anatomy is concave.

However, if the bone on the facial or lingual alveolar crest is thicker than normal, pressure can be placed in that direction. Still, it is important to realize that when applying pressure coronally in a lateral direction toward the alveolar crest, the apical portion of the tooth will be forced against the opposite socket wall. This pressure can lead to fracture of the apex, leaving a root tip to retrieve (Fig 6-10). Mandibular bone is denser than maxillary bone; therefore, root fracture is more probable in the mandible, depending on the root anatomy.

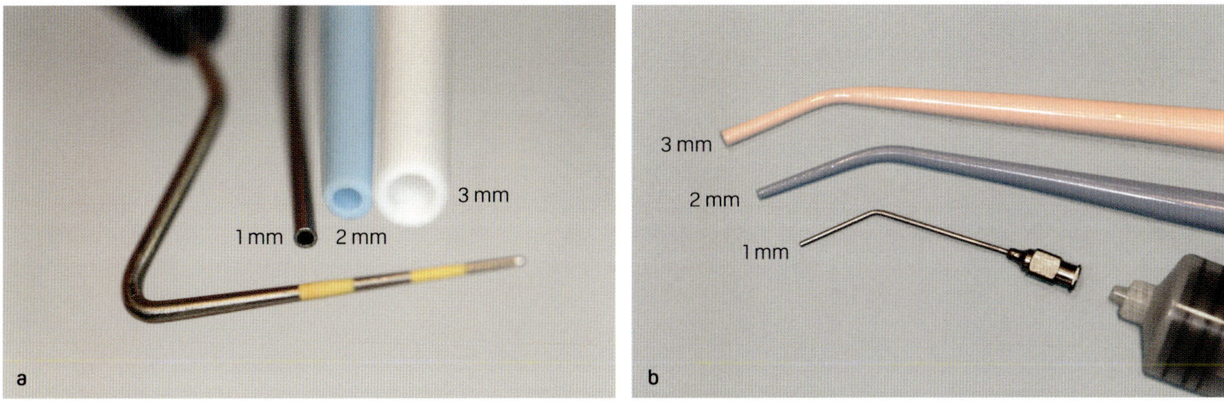

FIG 6-11 *(a and b)* Thin 1-mm irrigation tip and 2- and 3-mm-diameter suction tips used during sectioning of a crown.

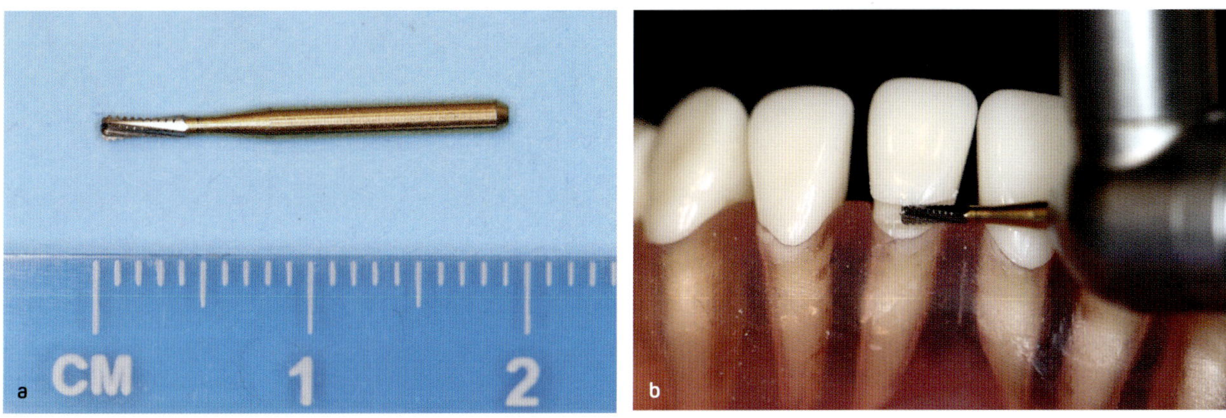

FIG 6-12 *(a)* Great White crosscut fissure bur used to horizontally section the crown. *(b)* Sectioning the mandibular right central incisor 1 mm coronal to the free gingival margin.

If there is a full-coverage restoration, luxation may or may not remove the crown. If gentle luxation is not successful in removing the tooth, the crown (whether a cemented full-coverage restoration or natural tooth) should be sectioned horizontally about 1 mm coronal to the gingival margin as described in the next section.

Section Crown Horizontally at the Cementoenamel Junction

Some practitioners remove the crown as the first step for every extraction, feeling that it is the most efficient and atraumatic method.

When sectioning a crown or roots, it is important to use plenty of saline irrigation with a thin irrigation tip to remove tooth debris and to use thin suction tips to suction within the drill cuts (Fig 6-11). This allows you to see and feel in these areas. Section the crown 1 mm coronal to the gingival margin using a Great White (SS White) high-speed crosscut fissure bur (Fig 6-12). It is important to be aware of the gingival margin location to avoid lacerating the gingiva.

Obviously, it's much easier to section through tooth structure or a composite restoration as compared to a metal restoration. Regardless of the material, section two-thirds of the way through the crown, and then, using an elevator, gently pry off the crown. Using a football-shaped diamond bur, smooth the remaining tooth structure to create a fairly flat surface approximately 1 mm coronal to the gingival margin (Fig 6-13).

Removing the crown allows you to see the remaining root structure anatomy and determine the best location to section vertically. Vertical fractures may be evident also. A dye such as To Dye For (Roydent) may be used to help visualize possible fractures.

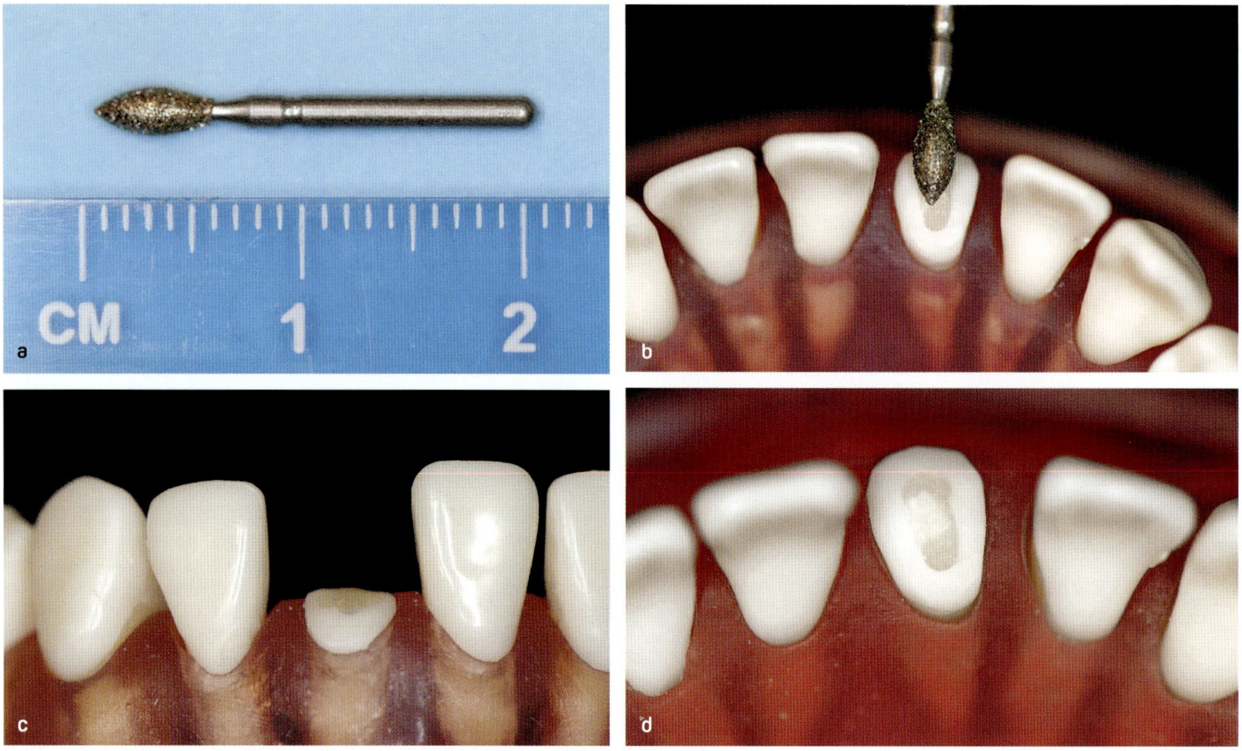

FIG 6-13 *(a and b)* Football diamond bur used to smooth the remaining root to a level 1 mm above the gingival margin after sectioning off the crown. *(c and d)* Occlusal and facial views of the mandibular right central incisor sectioned horizontally 1 mm above the gingival margin.

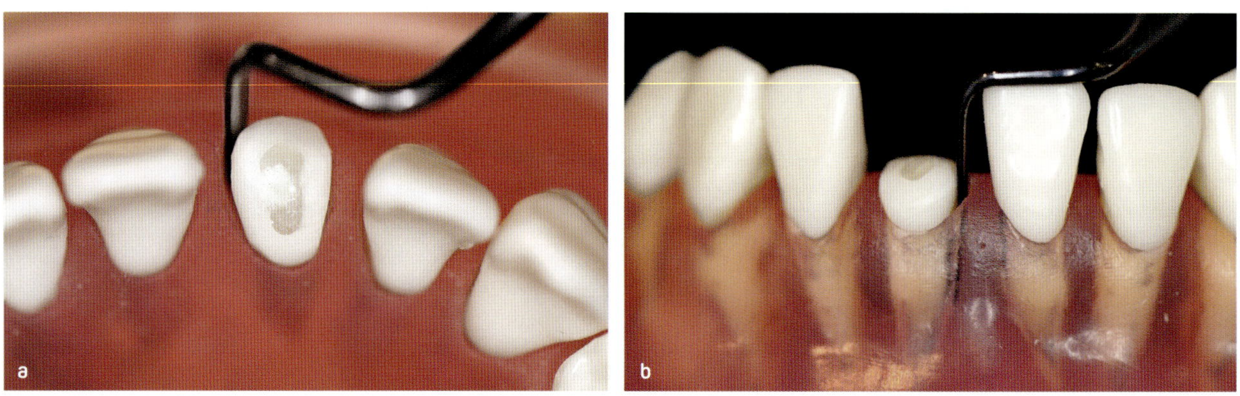

FIG 6-14 *(a and b)* Periotome in the sulcus using vertical pressure and a back-and-forth rocking motion. Avoid the facial, where the bone is thin.

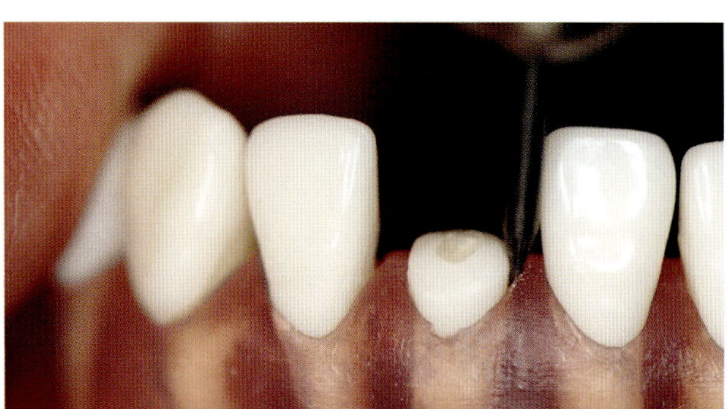

FIG 6-15 High-speed ¼ round bur used with a gentle up-and-down motion in the sulcus, exerting pressure toward the root, not the bone of the socket wall.

Optional procedure

Release the periodontal ligament fibers again using a narrow periotome (see Fig 6-4a). Enter the sulcus on the mesial, distal, and lingual, applying vertical pressure and a back-and-forth rocking motion to excise the periodontal ligament fibers further apically (Fig 6-14).

Recommended procedure

Instead of a periotome, you can use a ¼ round high-speed bur to further sever the periodontal ligament fibers (Fig 6-15). Attempt to cut more in the direction of the root rather than the bone of the socket wall. Excising periodontal ligament fibers like this detaches the root from bone, allowing for easier extraction. Avoid the facial aspect because bone in this area is thin.

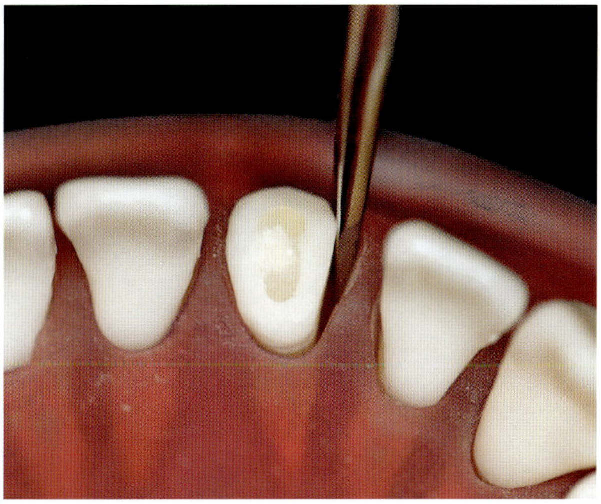

FIG 6-16 A thin Hu-Friedy EL3C elevator is used to gently luxate the root with a twisting motion, attempting to elevate it out of the socket.

Use Thin Elevator to Attempt Root Removal Coronally Without Flap Reflection

Introducing a thin elevator (see Fig 6-6a) at the mesiofacial and distofacial, use a twisting motion to attempt to move the root coronally (Fig 6-16). If the root moves but not coronally, release the periodontal ligament fibers again with the periotome or surgical-length high-speed ¼ round bur, then try the elevators again at the mesiofacial and distofacial. If you are not able to remove the root at this point, the next step is to insert the beaks of an incisor forceps as apically as possible and attempt luxation and slight rotation one more time (Fig 6-17).

If this is not successful, the next step is to vertically section the root.

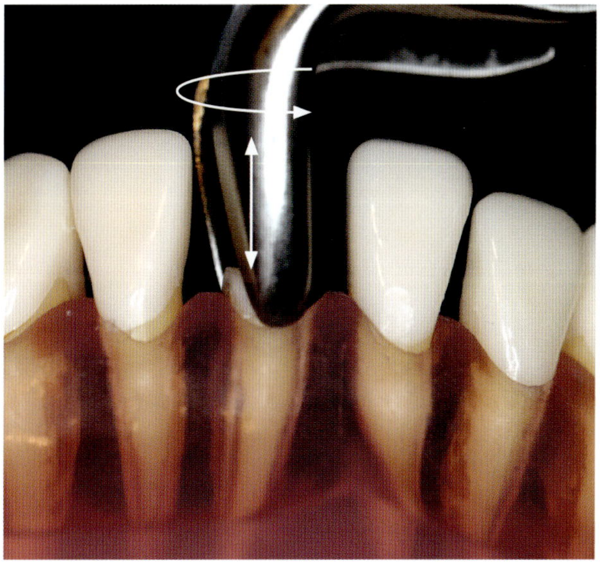

FIG 6-17 Using an incisor forceps to mobilize the mandibular right central incisor root.

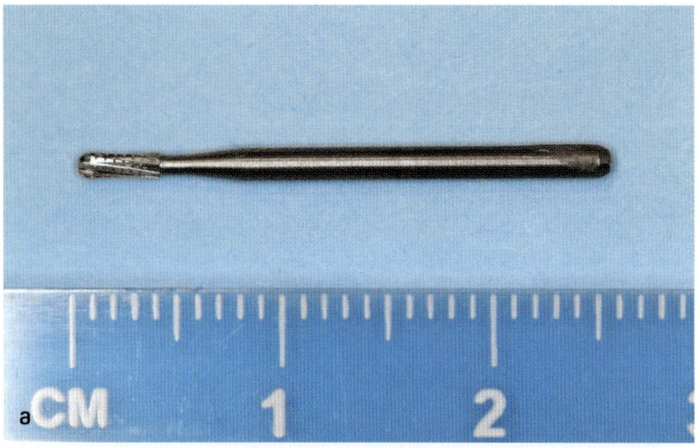

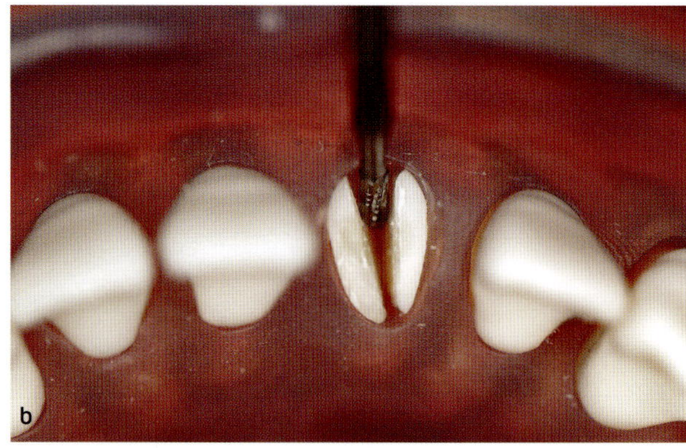

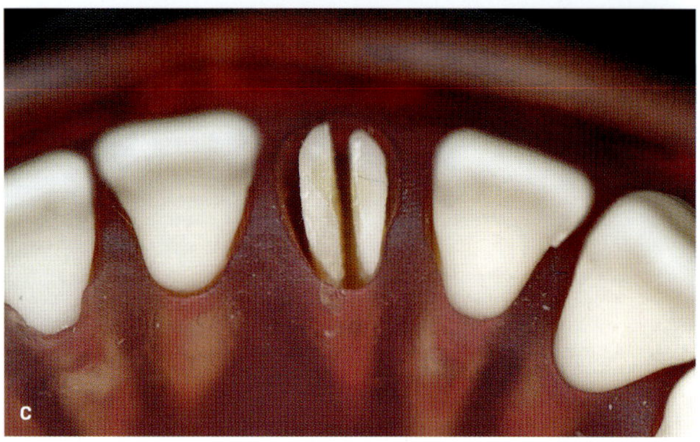

FIG 6-18 *(a)* Surgical-length high-speed crosscut fissure bur. *(b)* The bur is used to create space into which the root halves can be pressured (RSCET). *(c)* The mandibular right central incisor root sectioned vertically in a faciolingual direction.

Section Roots Vertically

This technique is termed the *root space creation extraction technique* (*RSCET*). The concept involves using a surgical-length high-speed crosscut fissure bur to remove tooth structure, creating a space into which the root can be pressured, away from the sulcus and socket wall (Fig 6-18a). In this way, a tooth can be removed without removing supporting bone. Single-rooted teeth usually are sectioned in a faciolingual direction so that mobilization of the root fragments does not stress the facial bone, but care must be taken to avoid scoring the facial bone (Figs 6-18b and 6-18c). This concept applies for the mandibular canines, but since the mandibular incisors are very thin mesiodistally, you may have to section in a mesiodistal direction. Also, since the mandibular anterior tooth roots are so narrow, a smaller round bur may be necessary. It is important that you have thin sterile saline irrigation and suction tips that reach the apices of the roots you are sectioning, allowing you to irrigate and suction the drill cuts, removing tooth debris for visualization.

Verify the location of the mental foramen and mandibular canal. Be aware of the submental and sublingual arteries lingual to the lingual plate in the floor of the mouth. Be careful to avoid these anatomical structures when sectioning and luxating these teeth.

If the root is not sectioned entirely through the apex, pressuring the root into the space may result in a horizontal fracture at the depth of the cut (Fig 6-19a). Therefore, if the surgical-length high-speed crosscut fissure bur does not reach the apex, use a straight handpiece round bur #4 or #6 to complete cutting through the apex. This requires opening up the cut wider at the coronal aspect to allow room for the shank of the straight handpiece bur (Figs 6-19b and 6-19c). When you feel the bur "drop" into the softer bone, you know you have sectioned completely through the apex (Fig 6-19d). Cut toward the lingual and facial slightly to make sure the cut is entirely through the root structure.

Once you have confirmed that the root has been completely divided through the apex, proceed as follows.

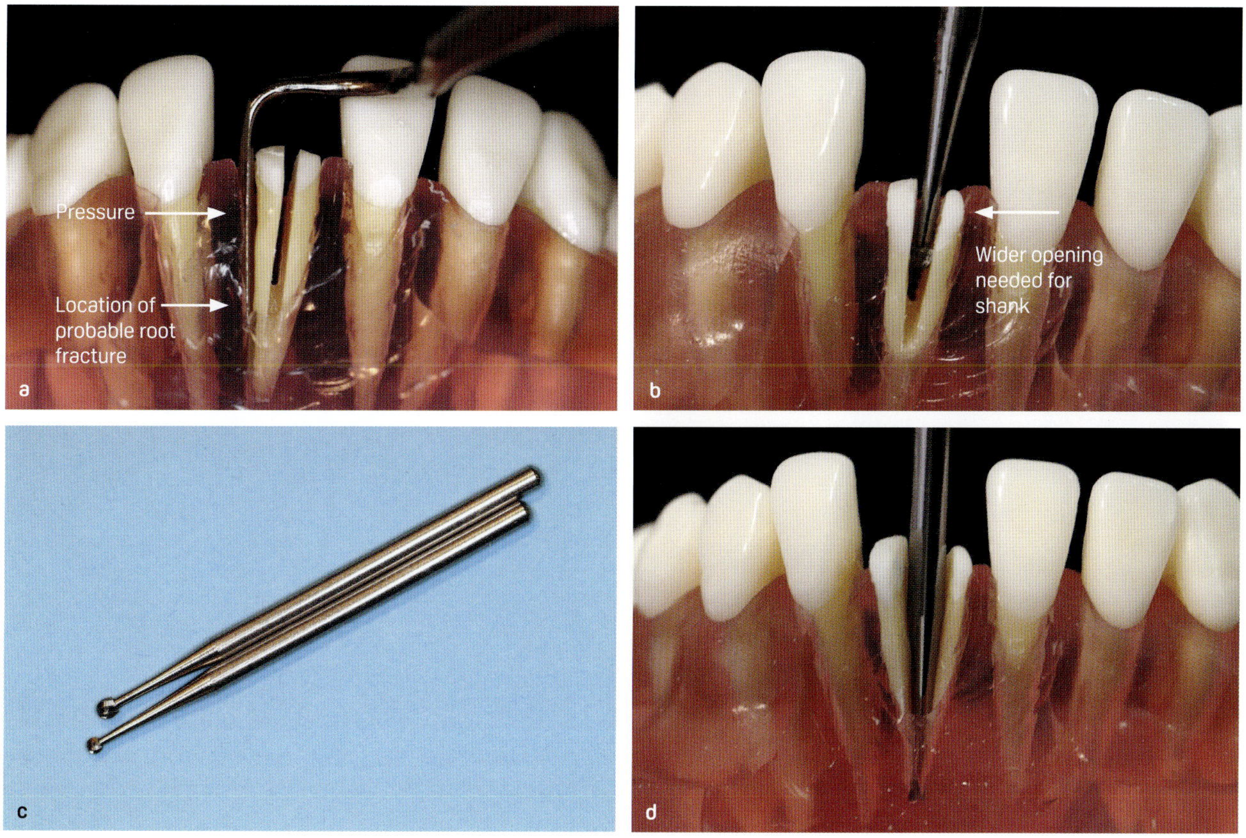

FIG 6-19 *(a)* Orban knife at the distal of the mandibular right central incisor, pressuring the incompletely sectioned root. There is a risk of fracturing the root at the depth of the cut, leaving the apex attached to the remaining root (gingiva removed for visualization purposes). *(b)* Root not sectioned entirely through apex. A wider opening is needed to allow room for the shank of the straight handpiece bur. *(c)* Straight handpiece burs #6 *(top)* and #4 *(bottom)*; the smaller bur (#4) is used for smaller roots, and #6 is used for larger roots. *(d)* Straight handpiece bur #4 sectioning completely past the apex into bone.

Elevate Gently Between Sectioned Root Pieces

Enter the sectioned space with a thin Directa L2S or Hu-Friedy EL3C elevator and gently pressure the root fragments laterally using a twisting motion (Fig 6-20). Be aware that you are also pressuring the bone laterally, so if it looks like there is a weak area of bone, avoid pressuring that area.

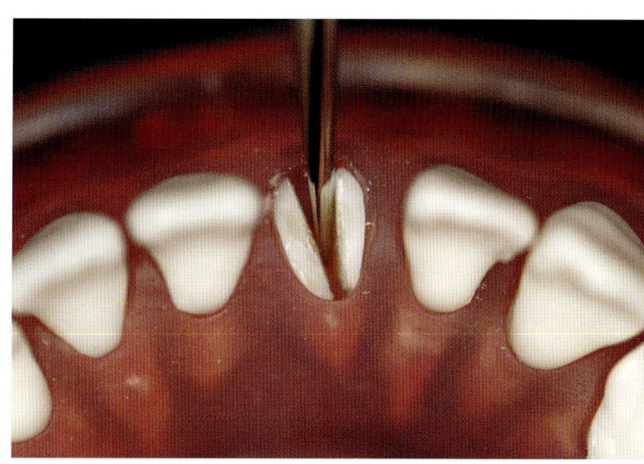

FIG 6-20 Thin elevator used with a gentle twisting motion to pressure root sections laterally.

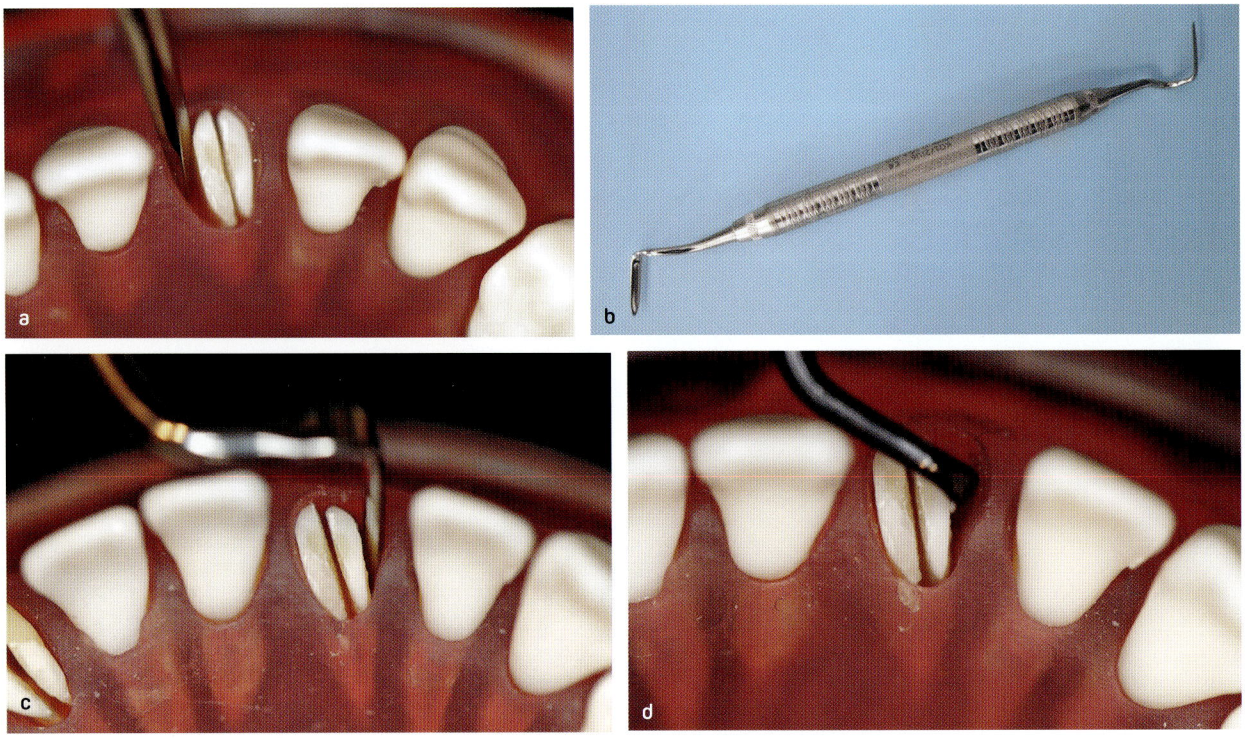

FIG 6-21 Various instruments used with vertical pressure and a back-and-forth rocking motion to pressure the root halves inward, into the space created by sectioning of the root (RSCET). *(a)* Thin Hu-Friedy EL3C elevator. *(b and c)* Hu-Friedy Orban knife KO1/2IU. *(d)* Periotome.

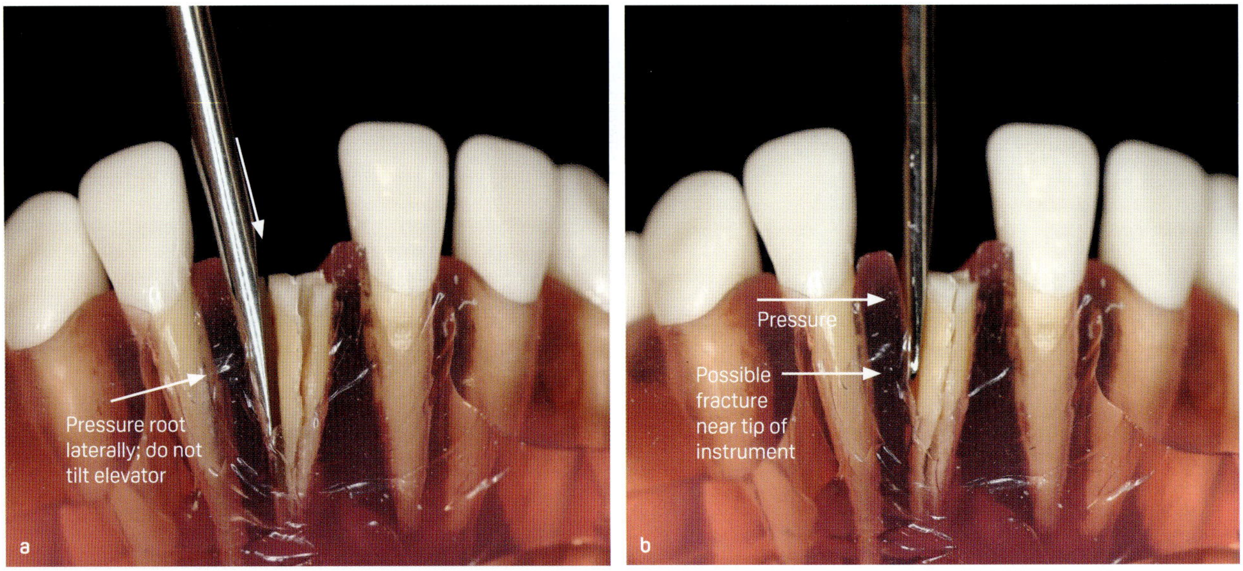

FIG 6-22 *(a)* Placement of the thin elevator as far apically as possible in the periodontal ligament space to pressure, rather than tilt, the root. *(b)* If the thin elevator is positioned only halfway down the root surface, there is a greater chance the root will fracture as it is pressured into the space created by sectioning the root. Pressure applied on the coronal half of the sectioned root stresses the mid-root area, leading to possible fracture, even if the root is fully sectioned through the apex.

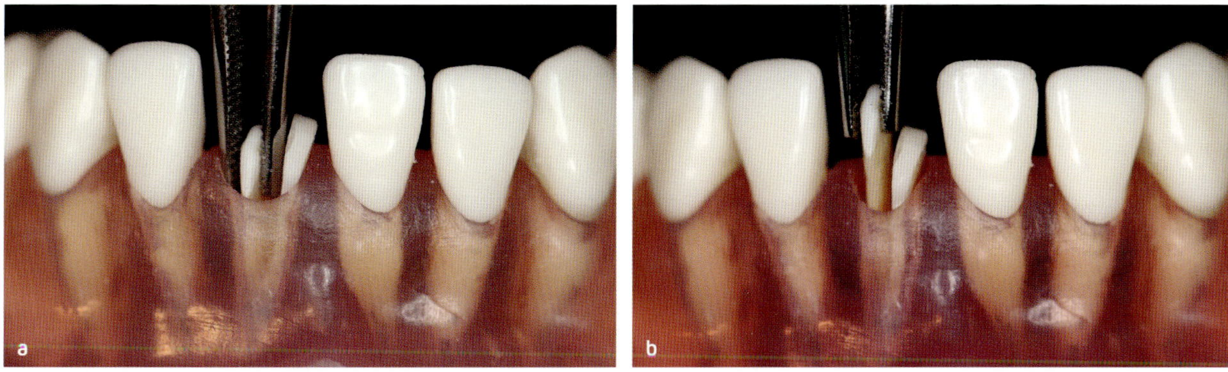

FIG 6-23 *(a)* Hemostat locked onto a mobile root segment. *(b)* A gentle back-and-forth motion with constant pulling pressure is used to remove the root segment from the socket.

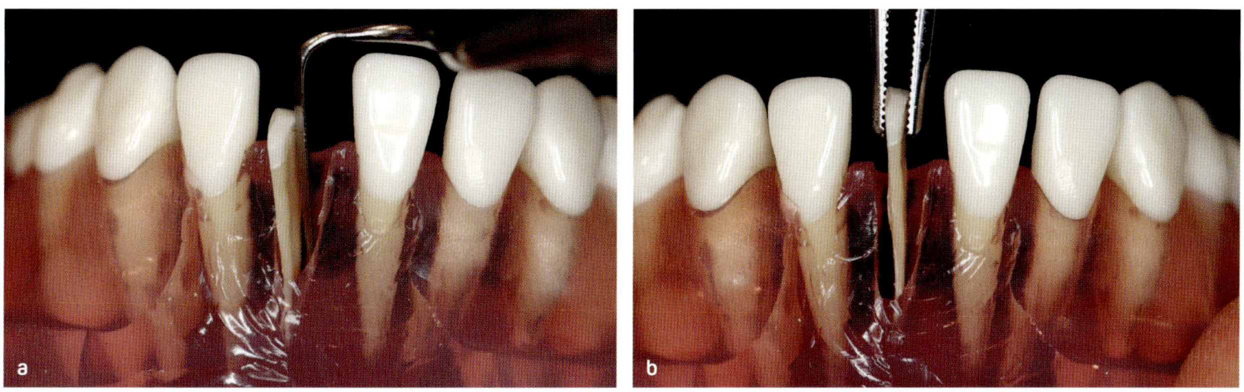

FIG 6-24 *(a)* Using an Orban knife to pressure the remaining root section into the space created when the initial half of the root was removed (RSCET). *(b)* Once this remaining root half has been mobilized into the root space, it can be removed with a hemostat or tweezers.

Enter Sulcus Laterally and Pressure Roots into Sectioned Space

Using an Orban knife, periotome, or thin elevator, enter the sulcus on the mesial and distal surfaces of the roots and attempt to force the root halves into the space created by sectioning the root (Fig 6-21). For the mandibular incisors, if they were sectioned mesiodistally, use the Orban knife or thin elevator at the mesiofacial or distofacial to push the roots into the space created by sectioning the roots. This will better protect the thin facial and lingual bone. It is important to make sure the instrument is seated as far apically as possible into the sulcus so the root is pressured horizontally rather than tilted, which may cause the root tip to fracture (Fig 6-22).

Be aware that you are pressuring against the adjacent bone, so do this in a gentle manner, paying attention to the integrity of the adjacent bone. As before, use thin irrigation and suction tips that reach the apex of the roots you are sectioning to irrigate and suction drill cuts. You may find that reentering the sectioned area and cutting between the root sections again may be required. If this does not mobilize the root fragments, it may be necessary to section the root fragments themselves (see next section).

Once root segments are mobilized, individual pieces can be removed with a hemostat. Lock a hemostat onto a mobile root segment as far apically as possible and use a gentle back-and-forth motion with constant pulling pressure to remove the root segment from the socket (Fig 6-23). This technique is helpful in many instances in which a tooth fragment has been mobilized and needs to be removed.

After one root section is removed, pressure the remaining root section into the space created by removal of the first (RSCET; Fig 6-24a). Then remove this second root half (Fig 6-24b).

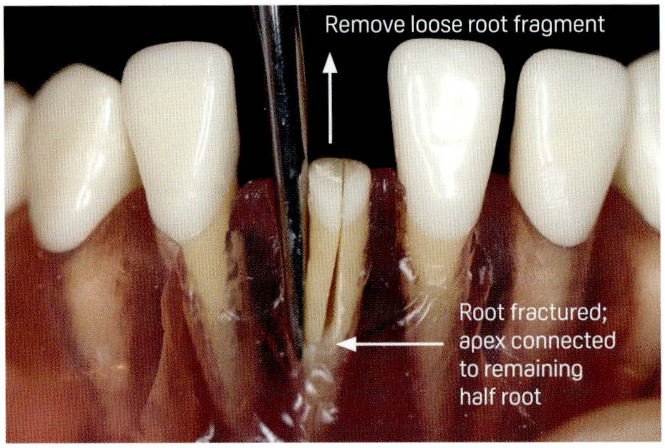

FIG 6-25 If horizontal fracture occurs, the first step is to remove the loose root fragment.

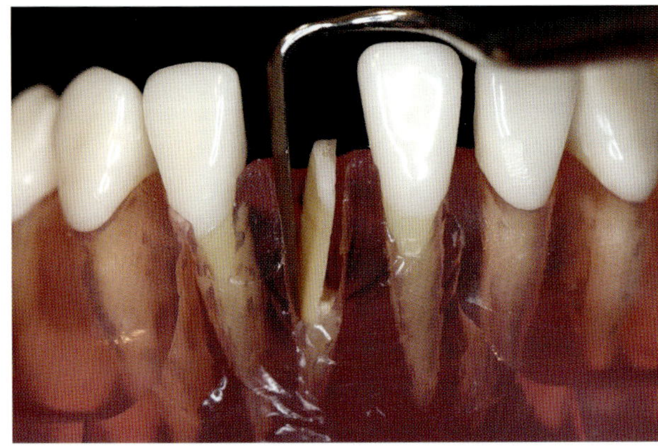

FIG 6-26 The Hu-Friedy Orban knife is used to pressure the remaining root, with apex attached, into the space created by removing the root fragment (RSCET).

Section Roots Again; Pressure into Space Created

If root halves cannot be mobilized and removed, consider vertically sectioning one and possibly both root halves so they are in quarters, being careful to avoid the mesial and distal socket walls. This is more applicable to larger roots, but smaller roots may require this step, at which time you are actually drilling out most of the root. Again, it is necessary to drill through the apex; feeling the bur drop into softer bone is an indication that you are past the apex. Then, pressure those root quarters into the space created (RSCET) and remove them.

Once root removal is complete, proceed to socket debridement (see chapter 11).

Complications

If the root is not sectioned entirely through the apex or if the apex fractures, atraumatic removal is difficult. The following steps will help reduce the severity of such complications.

As mentioned earlier, if the root is not sectioned entirely through the apex, pressuring the root into the space may result in a horizontal fracture at the depth of the cut (see Fig 6-19a). If horizontal fracture occurs, remove the loose root fragment (Fig 6-25). The choice is then to attempt to pressure the remaining root, with the apex attached, into the space created by removing the root fragment or to section through the apex.

If the remaining root is pressured into the space created by removing the root fragment (RSCET; Fig 6-26), the risk is another horizontal root fracture, leaving the entire apex. This approach is more successful in softer maxillary bone. Attempting this in the denser mandibular bone will result in fractures more frequently. The other option is to section through the apex (Fig 6-27).

A fractured apex is a complication we will all experience. Sectioning entirely through the apex is necessary to help prevent these complications.

Once root removal is complete, proceed to socket debridement (see chapter 11).

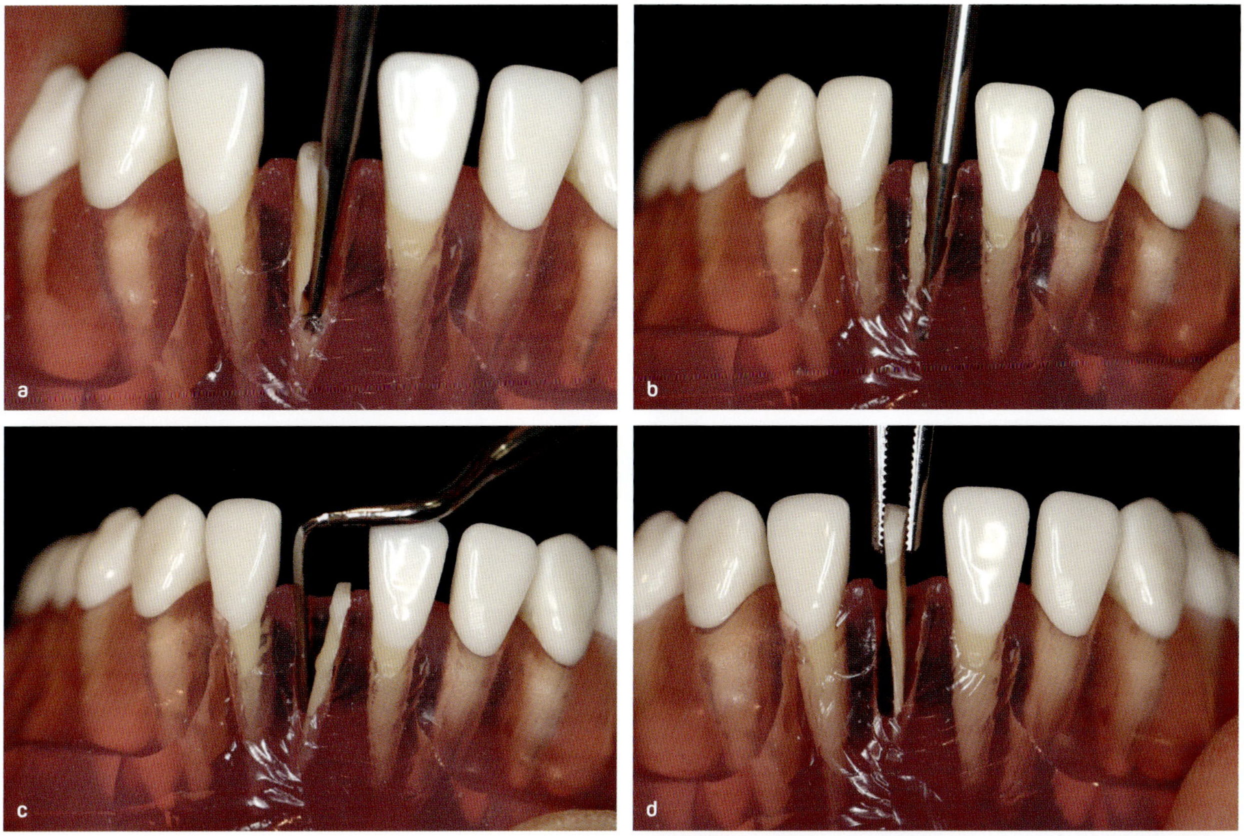

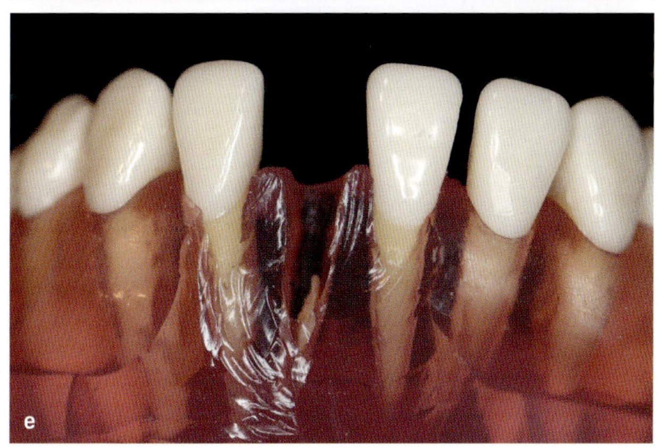

FIG 6-27 *(a and b)* If horizontal fracture occurs, remove the loose root fragment and use a straight handpiece bur #4 or #6 to completely section the root through the apex. *(c)* Once you are through the apex, use the Orban knife to pressure the root half into the space created by removal of the root fragment. *(d)* Remove the long root fragment. *(e)* Half apex remaining. This can be mobilized using a thin elevator and then removed with tweezers or by flushing with sterile saline.

7

Atraumatic Extraction of the Mandibular Premolars: Bone Is Dense

The following atraumatic extraction techniques apply to mandibular premolars with minimal to no mobility and good bone support. Obviously, teeth with Class II or III mobility can usually be removed atraumatically if there is adequate crown structure to grasp with a forceps. Also, it may not be necessary to use all of the following techniques to atraumatically remove a tooth. Some of the steps may be deemed nonproductive or not applicable to the clinical situation and therefore can be skipped at the discretion of the operating dentist.

The mandibular left second premolar is the demonstration example in this chapter; however, these principles apply to all mandibular premolars since they have similarly shaped roots.

Verify Profound Anesthesia

Probe the sulcus with a periodontal probe and stimulate adjacent gingiva, especially on the lingual, to confirm you have profound anesthesia (Fig 7-1). If anesthesia is inadequate, administer either another nerve block or infiltration into the sulcus and adjacent gingiva circumferentially (Fig 7-2). For quickest onset, use 4% articaine with 1:100,000 epinephrine. For hemostasis, 2% lidocaine 1:100,000 epinephrine is helpful.

A bite block can be used to stabilize the mandible; this also helps patients hold their mouth open during the procedure, reducing muscle fatigue.

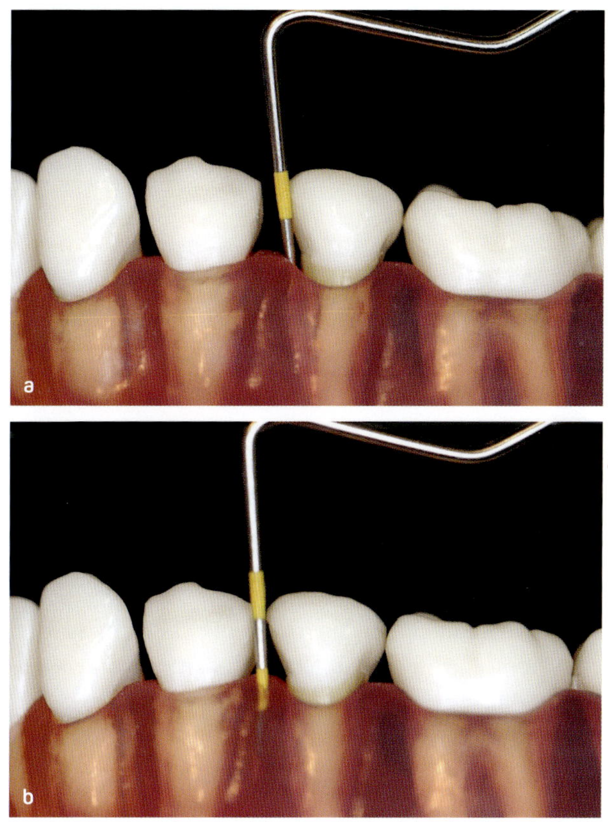

FIG 7-1 Verifying adequate anesthesia. *(a)* Probing the mesiobuccal sulcus of the mandibular left second premolar. *(b)* Probing the gingiva.

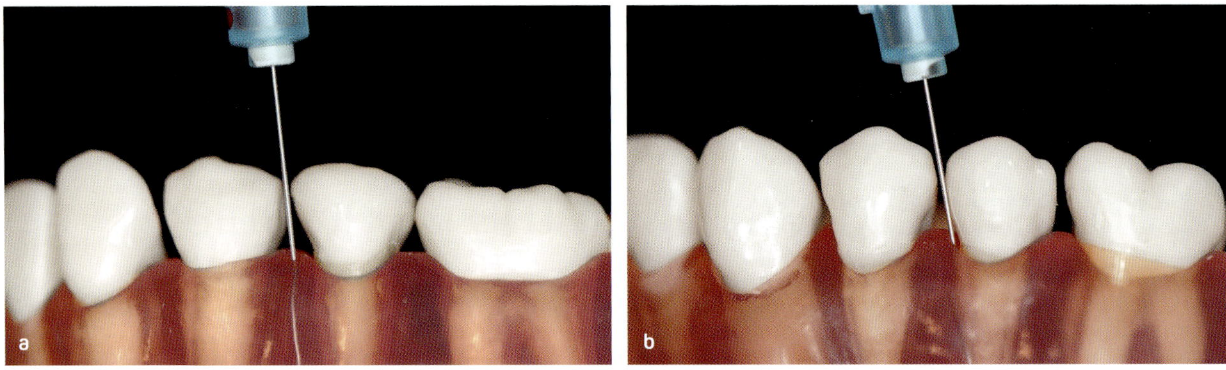

FIG 7-2 Supplementing anesthesia in adjacent gingiva and sulcus. *(a)* Infiltration into the papilla between the mandibular left first and second premolars. *(b)* Infiltration into the mesial sulcus of the mandibular left second premolar.

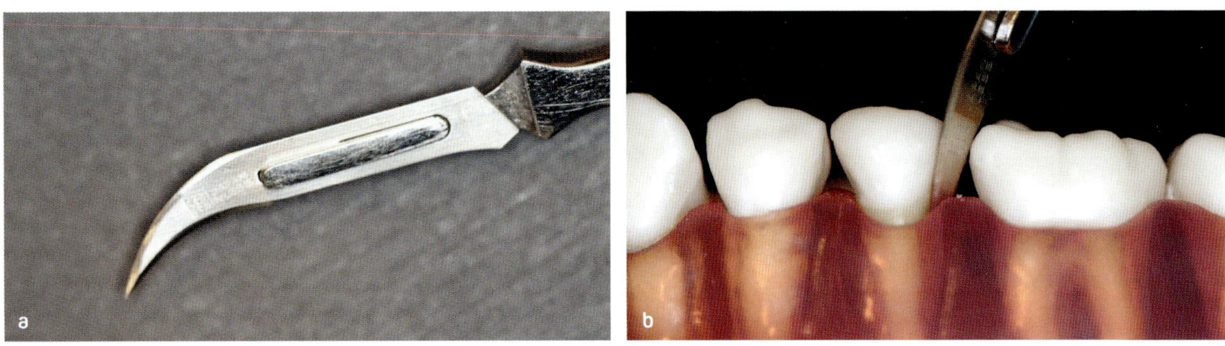

FIG 7-3 *(a)* A 12D scalpel blade. *(b)* The scalpel blade inserted into the distobuccal sulcus of the mandibular left second premolar to release the periodontal fibers using a back-and-forth rocking motion with vertical pressure.

Release Periodontal Ligament Fibers Without Flap Reflection

Note that some practitioners remove the crown as the first step. They feel that getting the crown out of the way and just dealing with the root(s) is the most efficient and atraumatic method to remove a tooth. For the purposes of this chapter, we will assume the crown will be left in place for these initial procedures.

Using a 12D scalpel blade, enter the sulcus on the mesial, distal, and lingual, but not the buccal due to the thin buccal bone being vulnerable to resorption and fracture. Apply vertical pressure with a back-and-forth rocking motion (Fig 7-3).

Optional procedure

Use a periotome to excise the periodontal ligament as deeply as possible two times in the mesial, distal, and lingual sulci (Fig 7-4). Use a back-and-forth motion with vertical pressure. However, it may be difficult to get into the periodontal ligament space due to lack of space or ankylosis. If that is the case, proceed to the recommended procedure below.

Recommended procedure

Use a ¼ round high-speed bur to further sever the periodontal ligament fibers (Fig 7-5a). Use an up-and-down pumping motion in the periodontal ligament space at the mesial, distal, and lingual, but avoid the buccal since the thin buccal bone is vulnerable to resorption and fracture (Fig 7-5b). Extend as far apically as possible, gently pressuring in the direction of the tooth root rather than the bone of the socket wall. This opening of the periodontal ligament space releases the tooth from the adjacent bone, making it easier to remove, and creates space for a thin elevator to enter and pressure the root.

A periotome, scalpel, or ¼ round high-speed bur can be used in any order.

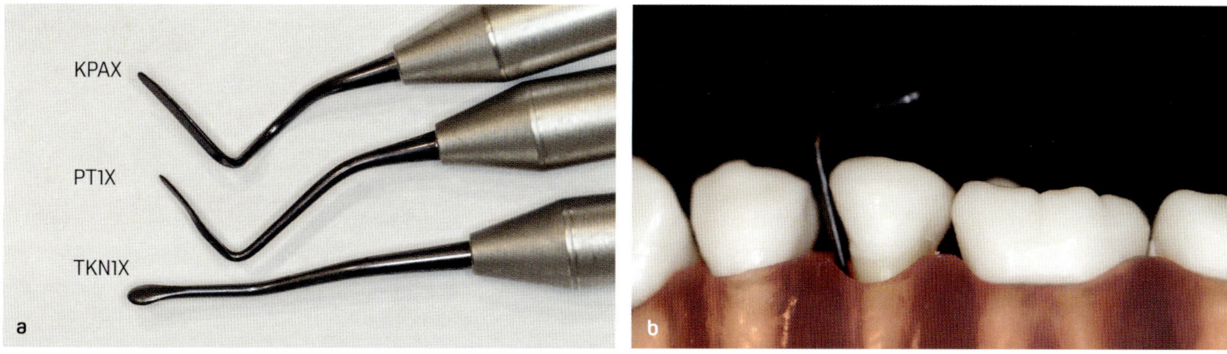

FIG 7-4 *(a)* Hu-Friedy periotomes. *(b)* Periotome inserted into the mesiobuccal sulcus of the mandibular left second premolar to excise the periodontal ligament fibers. Use vertical pressure and a back-and-forth rocking motion. Avoid the thin buccal bone.

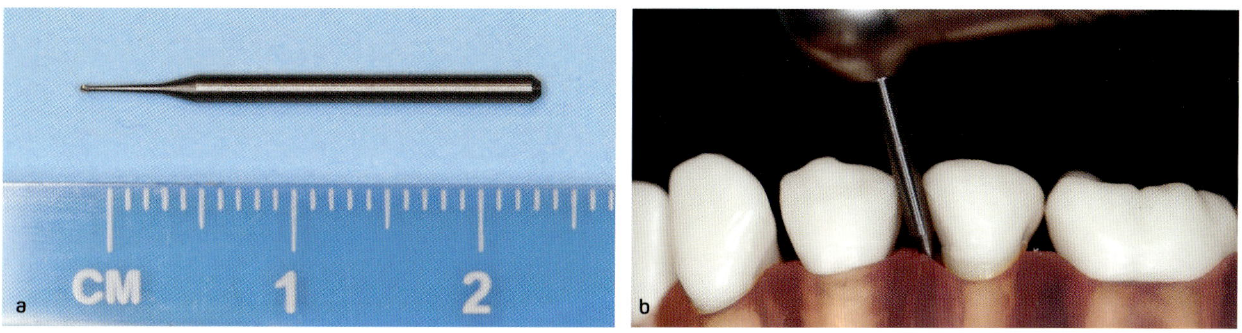

FIG 7-5 *(a)* Surgical-length ¼ round high-speed bur used to separate the root from the bone in the sulcus. *(b)* The bur is inserted in the sulcus with an up-and-down pumping motion with light pressure against the root, not the bone.

Attempt Tooth Removal Coronally Without Flap Reflection

Introduce a thin elevator (Fig 7-6) at the mesiobuccal and distobuccal and, using a twisting motion, attempt to move the tooth coronally (Fig 7-7).

At this point, if the tooth cannot be mobilized with a thin elevator or if there is not enough crown present to luxate the tooth but the root is intact, you can use the Easy X-Trac System (A. Titan) or Benex Root Extraction System (Meisinger) (see chapter 12). Both of these systems involve drilling a hole down the middle of the root canal space and inserting a threaded rod. This rod is pulled coronally with a wedging device, removing the root in one piece. To accomplish this, the crown must be cut horizontally approximately 1 mm above the gingival margin, being aware of the gingival margin location to avoid lacerating the gingiva. Since the root is tapered, there is minimal trauma when it is removed in a vertical direction with the Easy X-Trac or Benex. In my opinion, this is the most atraumatic method of removing a single-rooted tooth with a tapered root.

However, if there is adequate crown structure present for luxation of any kind, the following may be helpful.

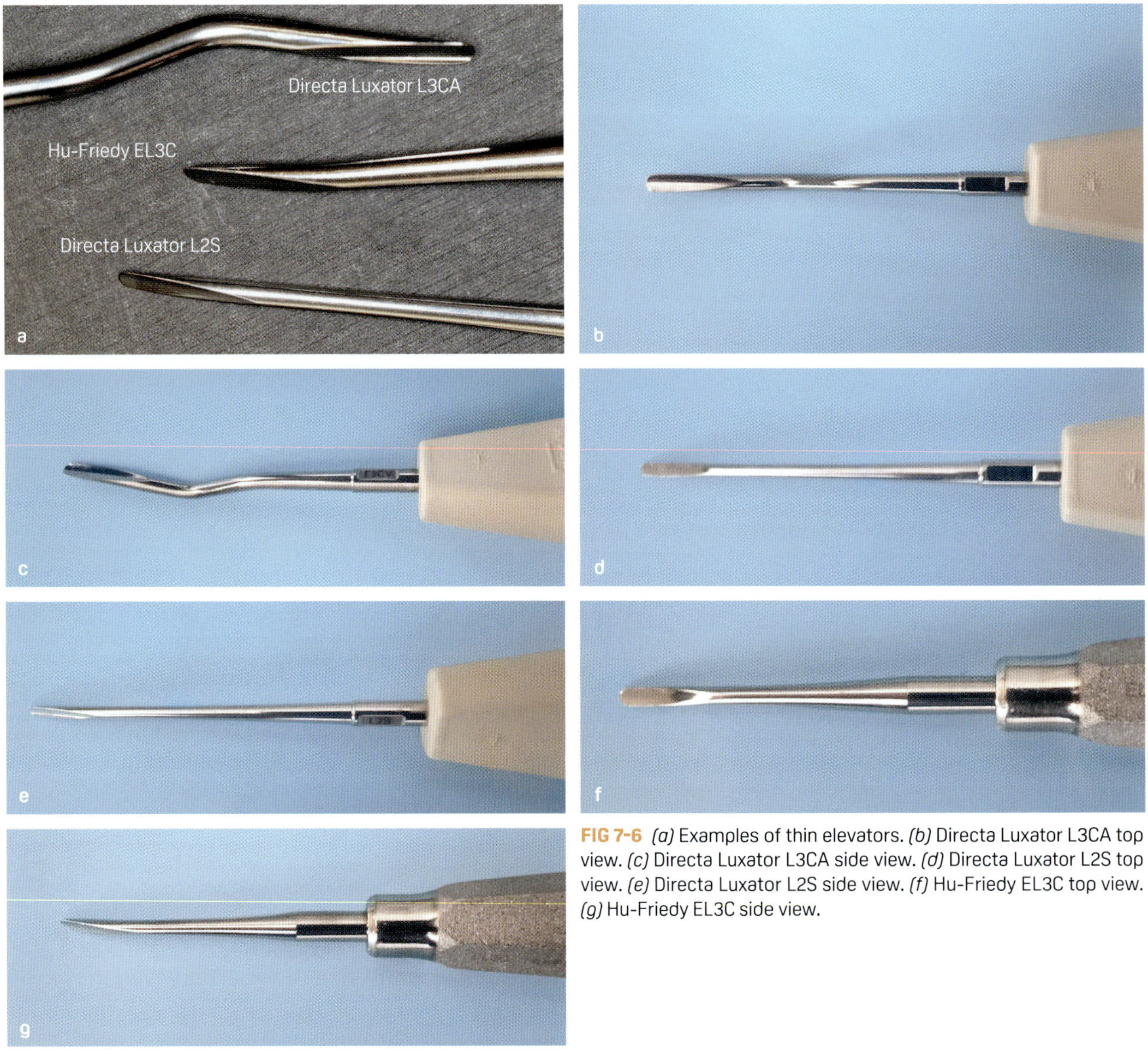

FIG 7-6 *(a)* Examples of thin elevators. *(b)* Directa Luxator L3CA top view. *(c)* Directa Luxator L3CA side view. *(d)* Directa Luxator L2S top view. *(e)* Directa Luxator L2S side view. *(f)* Hu-Friedy EL3C top view. *(g)* Hu-Friedy EL3C side view.

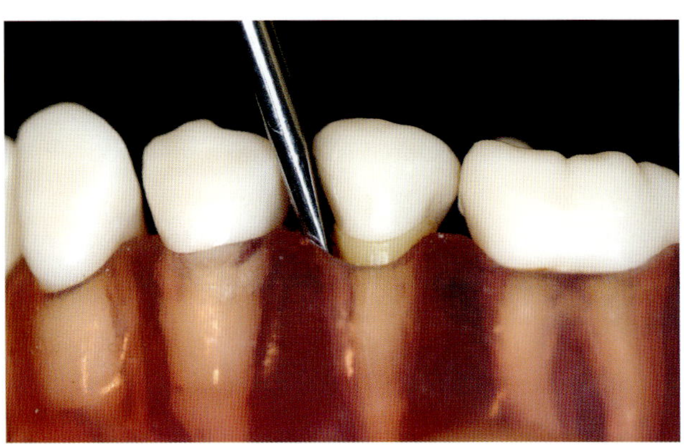

FIG 7-7 Thin elevator (Directa Luxator L2S) inserted at the mesiobuccal of the mandibular left second premolar.

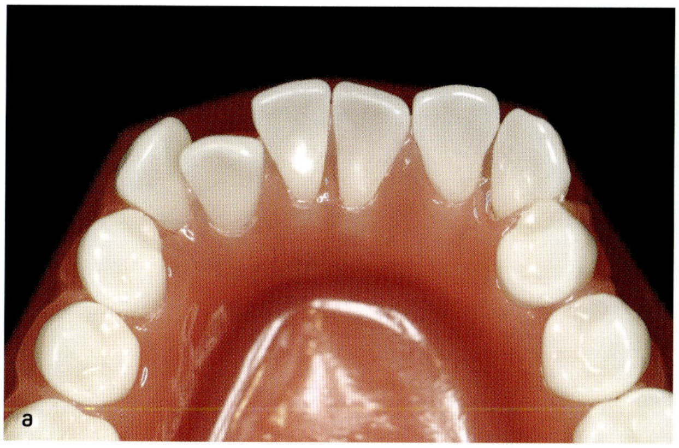

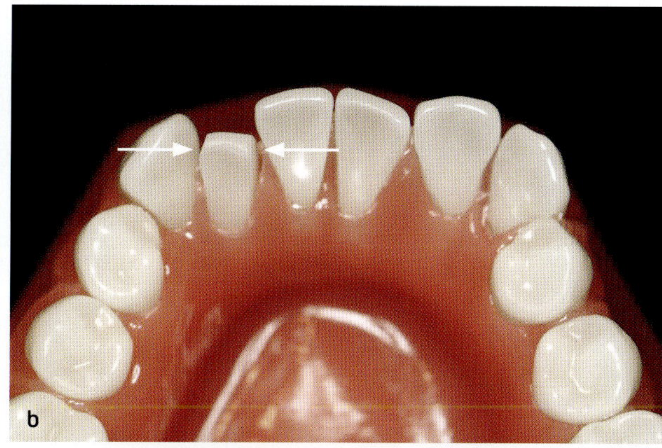

FIG 7-8 *(a)* Mandibular left lateral incisor overlapped with the adjacent canine and central incisor. Rotating the lateral incisor with a forceps will apply pressure to (and may cause increased mobility of) these adjacent teeth. *(b)* The mesial and distal contacts of the lateral incisor have been reduced. *(c)* Now rotation of the lateral incisor with a forceps will be less harmful to adjacent teeth.

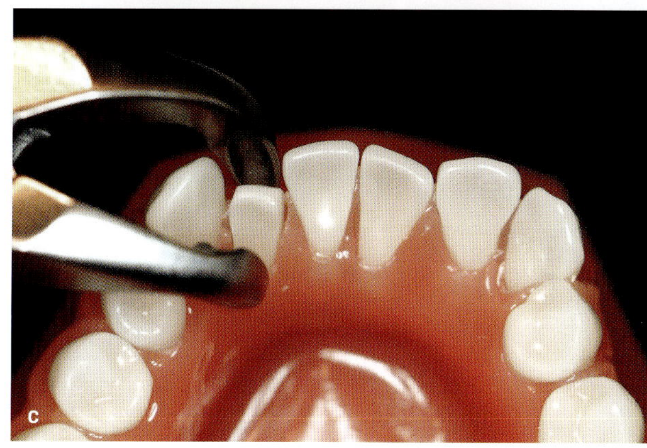

Reduce Interproximal Contacts

We are attempting to remove a tooth as atraumatically as possible, and this pertains not only to the tooth being extracted but also to the adjacent teeth, their restorations, and the rest of the mouth as well. If we were to rotate a tooth with tight or overlapping contacts, we would be pressuring the adjacent contacts and therefore moving the adjacent teeth. (If multiple adjacent teeth are being removed, this concept does not apply; luxation of a tooth with tight or overlapping contacts may actually help loosen adjacent teeth planned for extraction.) Therefore, where teeth are overlapped or crowded, I feel it is important to reduce the interproximal contacts on a single tooth to be removed. Note that if interproximal contacts are present, but luxation does not move or harm adjacent teeth or restorations, then reduction of interproximal contacts is not necessary. If contacts are overlapping on one side only, rotate the tooth in the direction that does not increase contact pressure. Figure 7-8 presents overlapping mandibular incisors as an example.

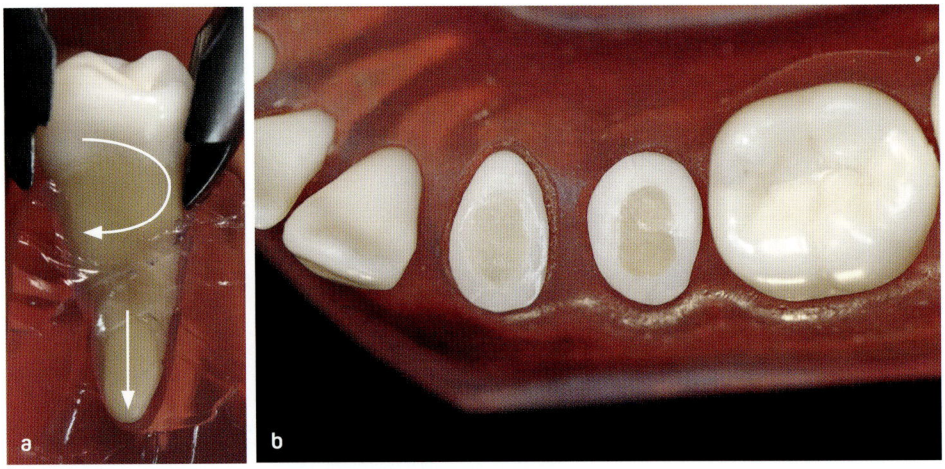

FIG 7-9 *(a)* Forceps applied as far apically as possible without damaging bone or soft tissue. First apply vertical pressure, then rotational movement. *(b)* Mandibular left first and second premolar roots with crowns removed to show anatomy.

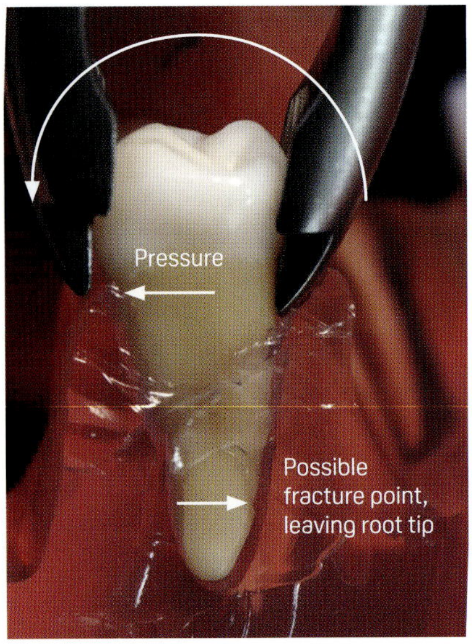

FIG 7-10 Pressure applied coronally toward the buccal of the mandibular left second premolar also pressures the lingual surface of the apex. This may result in a fracture of the apex.

Luxate Gently with Forceps

To gently luxate the tooth, place forceps as far apically as possible without engaging bone. Try to engage the root surface apical to any restoration margins. Gently apply pressure apically and hold for 30 seconds. While continuing to apply apical pressure, gently luxate in a twisting motion to test the mobility of the tooth (Fig 7-9a). The reason for applying apical pressure while luxating is that it shifts the axis of rotation in an apical direction, reducing the chance for root fracture. Remember that the roots of the mandibular premolars are oval in shape and much wider buccolingually than mesiodistally (Fig 7-9b). Rotating them will expand the socket and may fracture the socket wall.

If the bone on the buccal or lingual alveolar crest is especially thick, pressure can be placed in that direction. However, it is important to realize that when applying pressure coronally in a lateral direction toward the alveolar crest, the apical portion of the tooth will be forced against the opposite socket wall. This pressure can lead to fracture of the apex, leaving a root tip to retrieve (Fig 7-10). Mandibular bone is denser than maxillary bone; therefore, root fracture is more probable in the mandible, depending on the root anatomy.

If there is a full-coverage restoration, luxation may or may not remove the crown. If gentle luxation is not successful in removing the tooth, the crown (whether a cemented full-coverage restoration or natural tooth) should be sectioned horizontally about 1 mm coronal to the gingival margin as described in the next section.

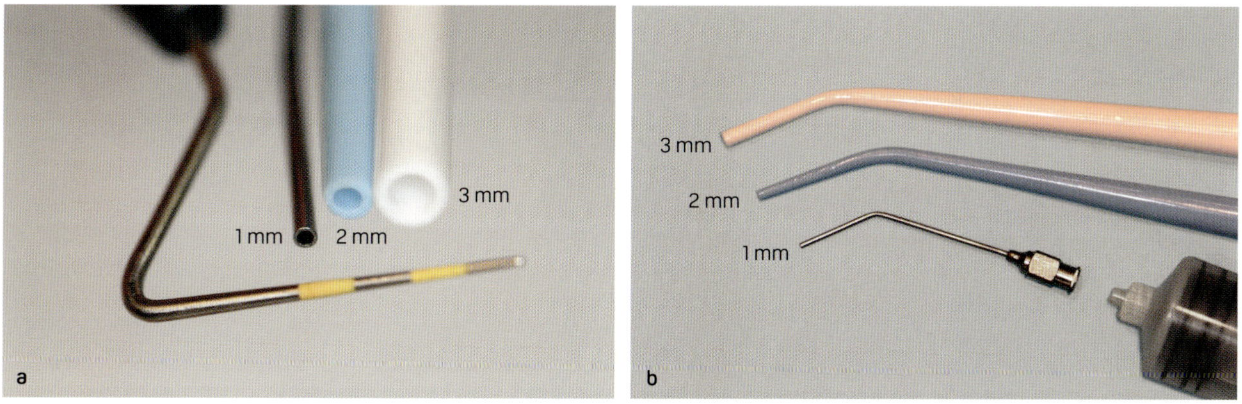

FIG 7-11 *(a and b)* Thin 1-mm irrigation tip and 2- and 3-mm-diameter suction tips used during sectioning of a crown.

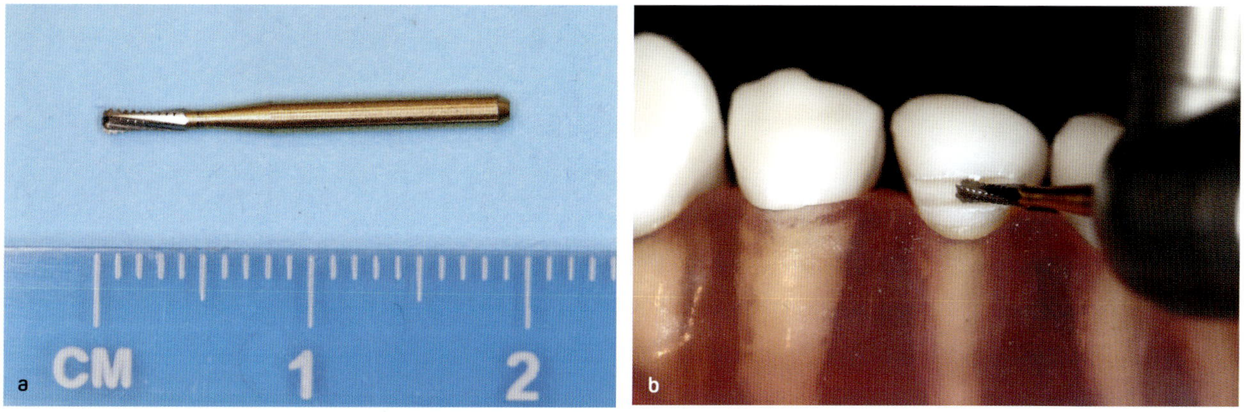

FIG 7-12 *(a)* Great White high-speed crosscut fissure bur used to horizontally section the crown. *(b)* Sectioning the mandibular left second premolar 1 mm coronal to the free gingival margin.

Section Crown Horizontally at the Cementoenamel Junction

Some practitioners go right to this step for every extraction, feeling that it is the most efficient and atraumatic method.

When sectioning a crown or roots, it is important to use plenty of saline irrigation with a thin irrigation tip to remove tooth debris and to use thin suction tips to suction within the drill cuts (Fig 7-11). This allows you to see and feel in these areas. Section the crown 1 mm coronal to the gingival margin using a Great White (SS White) high-speed crosscut fissure bur (Fig 7-12). It is important to be aware of the gingival margin location to avoid lacerating the gingiva.

Obviously, it's much easier to section through tooth structure or a composite restoration as compared to a metal restoration. Regardless of the material, section two-thirds of the way through the crown, and then, using an elevator, gently pry off the crown. Using a football-shaped high-speed diamond bur, smooth the remaining tooth structure to a fairly flat surface approximately 1 mm coronal to the gingival margin (Fig 7-13).

Removing the crown allows you to see the remaining root structure anatomy and determine the best location to section vertically. Vertical fractures may be evident also. A dye such as To Dye For (Roydent) may be used to help visualize possible fractures.

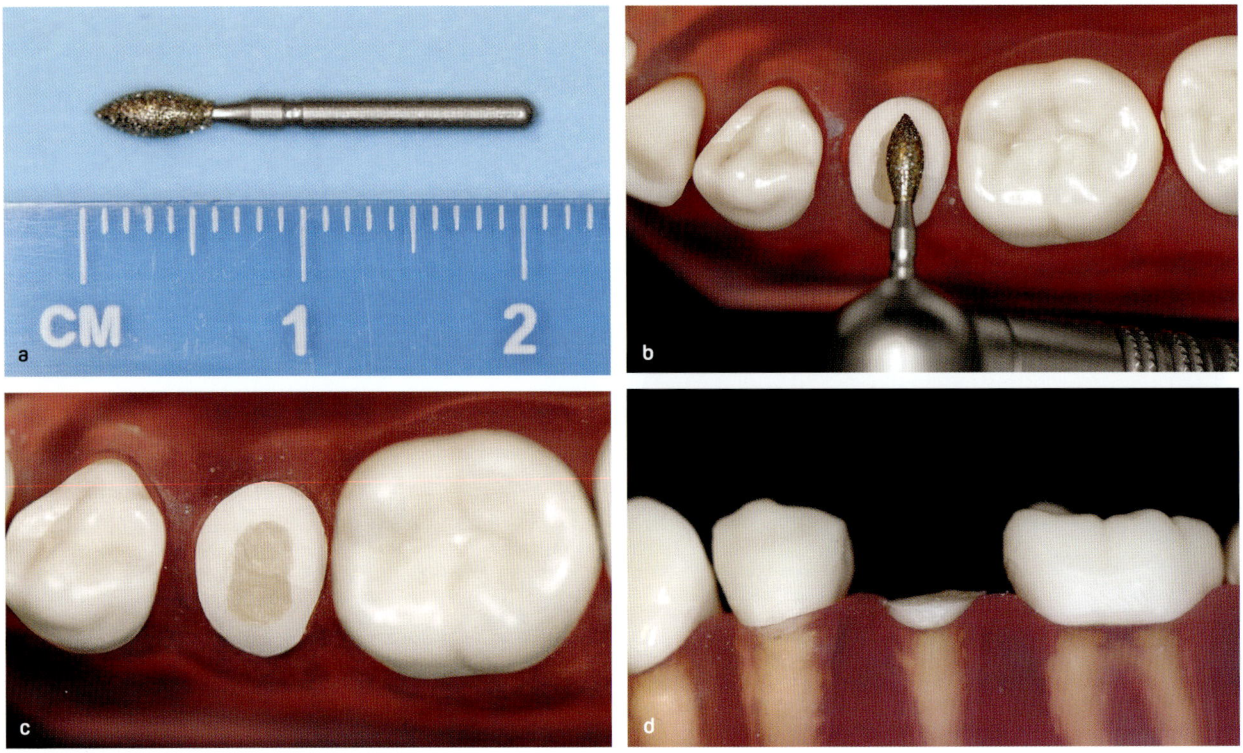

FIG 7-13 *(a and b)* High-speed football diamond bur used to smooth the remaining root to a level 1 mm above the gingival margin after sectioning off the crown. *(c and d)* Occlusal and buccal views of the mandibular left second premolar sectioned 1 mm coronal to the gingival margin.

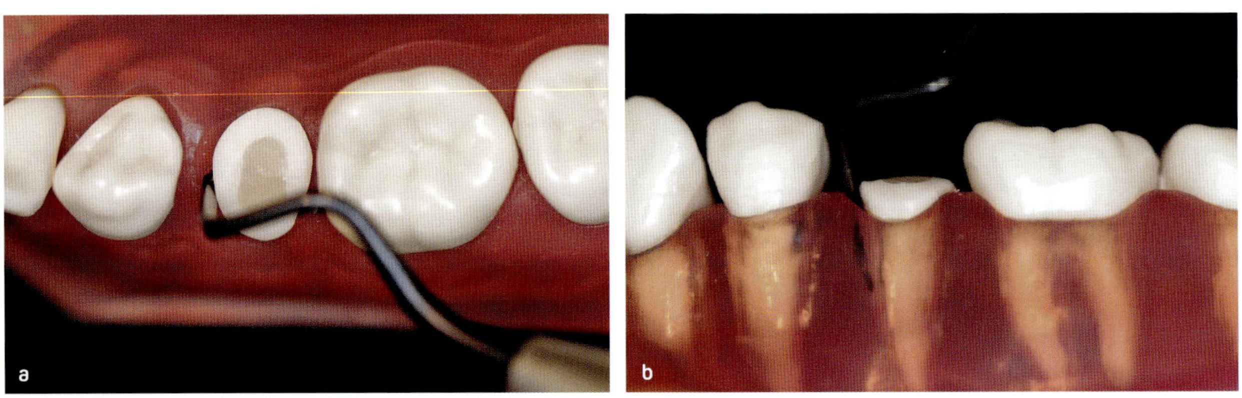

FIG 7-14 *(a and b)* Periotome in the sulcus using vertical pressure and a back-and-forth rocking motion. Avoid the buccal, where bone is thin.

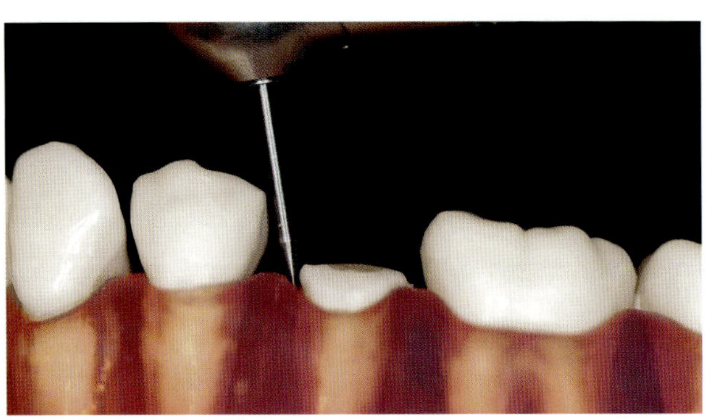

FIG 7-15 High-speed ¼ round bur used with a gentle up-and-down motion in the sulcus, exerting pressure toward the root, not the bone of the socket wall.

Optional procedure

Release the periodontal ligament fibers again using a narrow periotome (see Fig 7-4a). Enter the sulcus on the mesial, distal, and lingual, applying vertical pressure and a back-and-forth rocking motion to excise the periodontal ligament fibers further apically (Fig 7-14).

Recommended procedure

Instead of a periotome, you can use a high-speed ¼ round bur to further sever the periodontal ligament fibers (Fig 7-15). Attempt to cut more in the direction of the root rather than the bone of the socket wall. Excising periodontal ligament fibers like this detaches the root from bone, allowing for easier extraction. Avoid the buccal aspect because bone in this area is thin.

Use Thin Elevator to Attempt Root Removal Coronally Without Flap Reflection

Introducing a thin elevator (see Fig 7-6a) at the mesiobuccal and distobuccal, use a twisting motion to attempt to move the root coronally (Fig 7-16). If the root moves but not coronally, release the periodontal ligament fibers again with the periotome or high-speed ¼ round bur, then try the elevators again at the mesiobuccal and distobuccal. If you are not able to remove the root at this point, the next step is to insert the beaks of an incisor forceps as apically as possible and attempt luxation and slight rotation one more time (Fig 7-17).

If this is not successful, the next step is to vertically section the root.

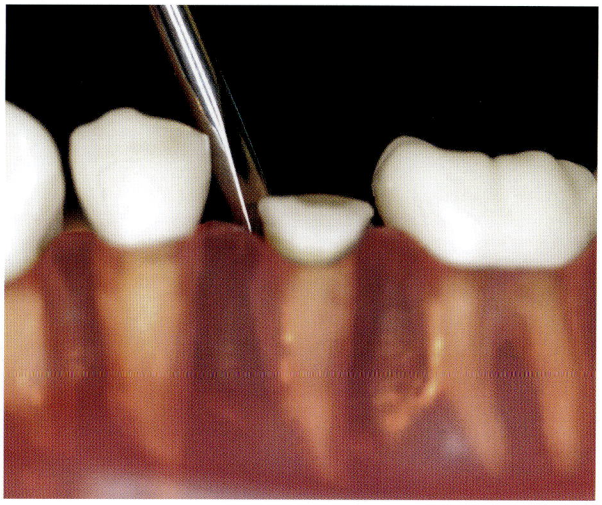

FIG 7-16 A thin Hu-Friedy EL3C elevator is used to gently luxate the root with a twisting motion, attempting to elevate it out of the socket.

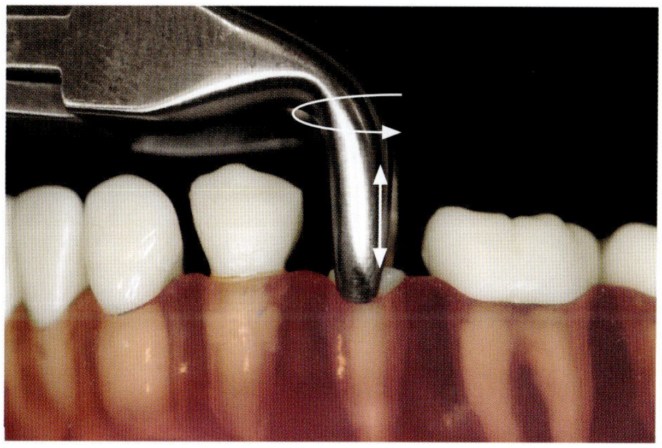

FIG 7-17 Using an incisor forceps to mobilize the mandibular left second premolar root.

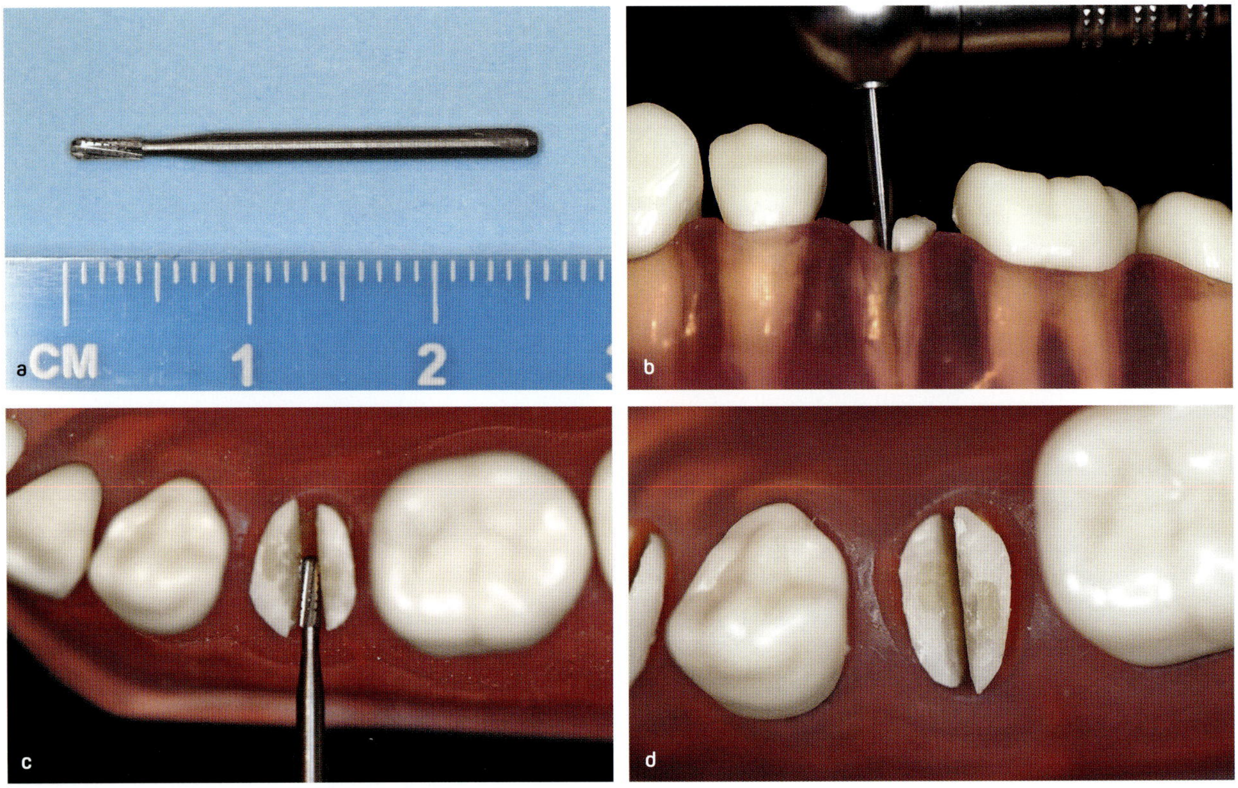

FIG 7-18 *(a)* Surgical-length high-speed crosscut fissure bur. *(b and c)* The bur is used to section the root buccolingually, creating space into which the root halves can be pressured (RSCET). *(d)* The mandibular left second premolar sectioned vertically in a buccolingual direction.

Section Roots Vertically

This technique is termed the *root space creation extraction technique* (*RSCET*). The concept involves using a surgical-length high-speed crosscut fissure bur to remove tooth structure and creating a space into which the root can be pressured, away from the sulcus and socket wall (Fig 7-18a). In this way, a tooth can be removed without removing supporting bone. Single-rooted teeth, including the mandibular premolars, are usually sectioned in a buccolingual direction so that mobilization of the root fragments does not stress the buccal bone, but care must be taken to avoid scoring the buccal bone (Figs 7-18b to 7-18d). It is important that you have thin sterile saline irrigation and suction tips that reach the apices of the roots you are sectioning, allowing you to irrigate and suction the drill cuts, removing tooth debris for visualization.

Verify the location of the mental foramen and mandibular canal. Be aware of the submental and sublingual arteries lingual to the lingual plate in the floor of the mouth. Be careful to avoid these anatomical structures when sectioning and luxating these teeth.

If the root is not sectioned entirely through the apex, pressuring the root into the space may result in a horizontal fracture at the depth of the cut (Fig 7-19a). Therefore, if the surgical-length high-speed crosscut fissure bur does not reach the apex, use a straight handpiece round bur #4 or #6 to complete cutting through the apex. This requires opening up the cut wider at the coronal aspect to allow room for the shank of the straight handpiece bur (Figs 7-19b and 7-19c). When the root is completely sectioned through the apex, you will feel your handpiece "drop" into the softer bone (Fig 7-19d). Cut toward the lingual and buccal slightly to make sure the cut is entirely through the root structure.

Once you have confirmed that the root has been completely divided through the apex, proceed as follows.

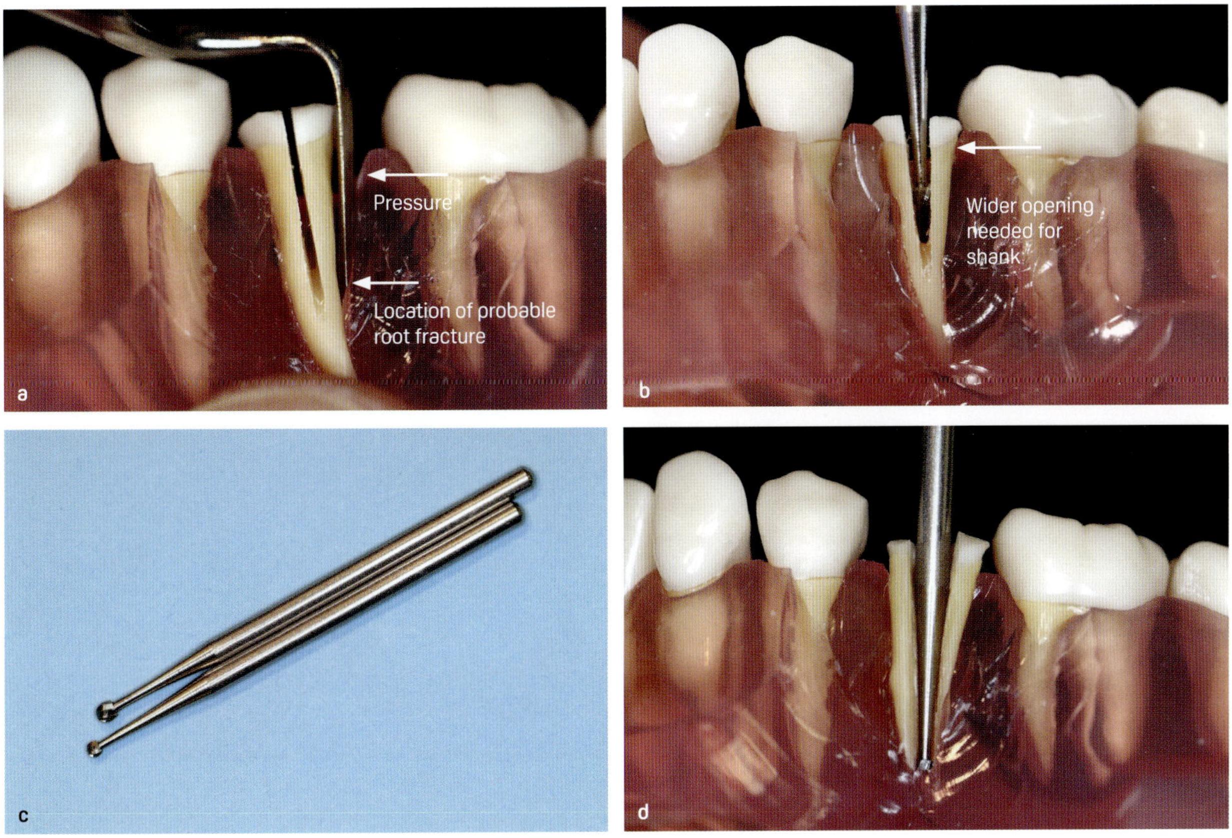

FIG 7-19 *(a)* Orban knife at the distal of the mandibular left second premolar, pressuring the incompletely sectioned root. There is a risk of fracturing the root at the depth of the cut, leaving the apex attached to the remaining root (gingiva removed for visualization purposes). *(b)* Root not sectioned entirely through apex. A wider opening is needed to allow room for the shank of the straight handpiece bur. *(c)* Straight handpiece burs #6 *(top)* and #4 *(bottom)*; the smaller bur (#4) is used for smaller roots, and #6 is used for larger roots. *(d)* Straight handpiece bur #4 sectioning completely past the apex into bone.

Elevate Gently Between Sectioned Root Pieces

Enter the sectioned space with a thin elevator and gently pressure the root fragments laterally using a twisting motion (Fig 7-20). Be aware that you are also pressuring the bone laterally, so if it looks like there is a weak area, avoid pressuring that area.

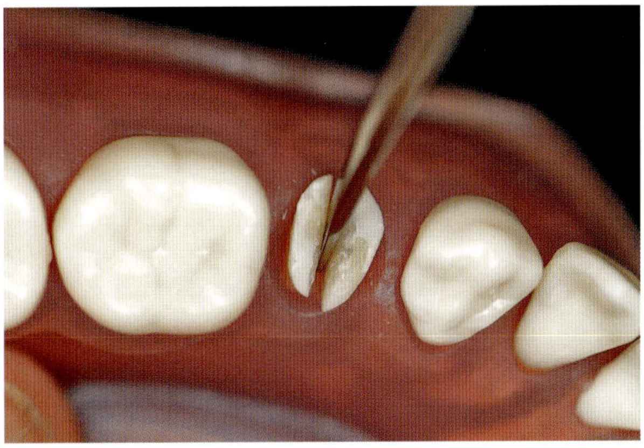

FIG 7-20 Thin Directa Luxator L2S elevator used with a gentle twisting motion to pressure root sections laterally.

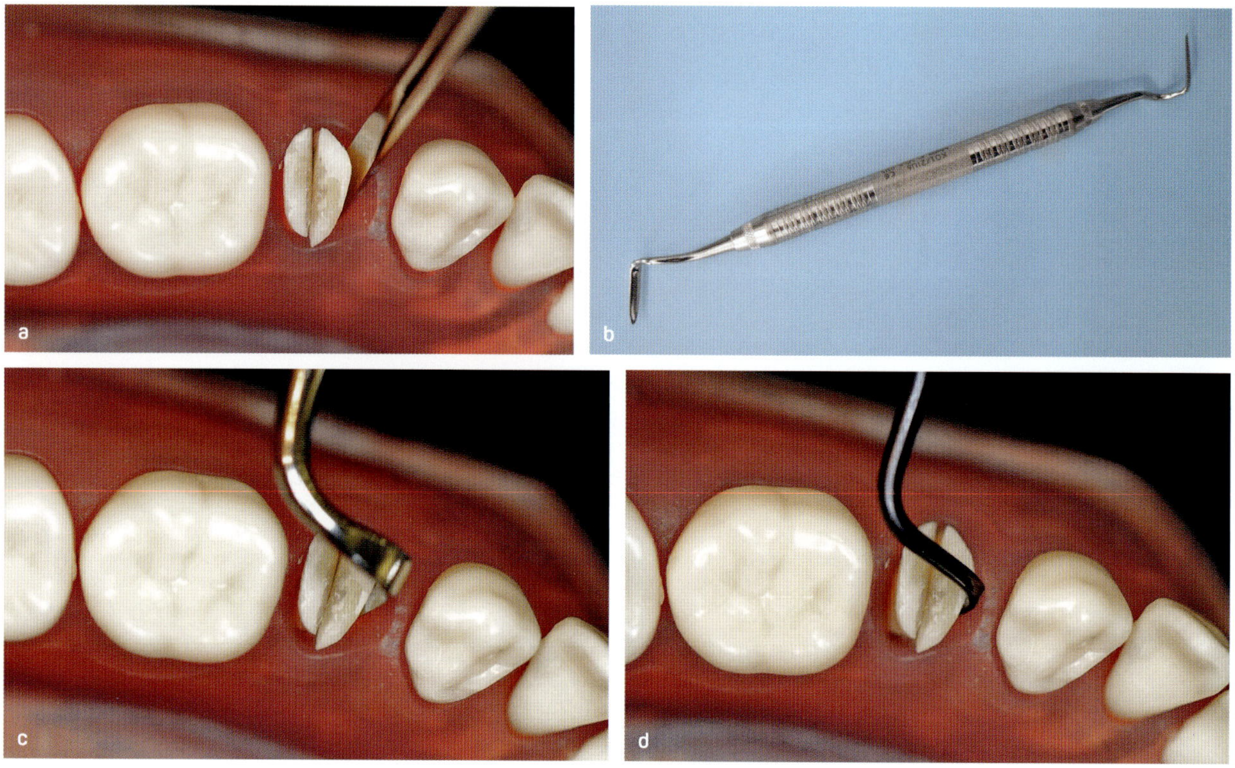

FIG 7-21 Various instruments used with vertical pressure and a back-and-forth rocking motion to pressure the root halves inward, into the space created by sectioning of the root (RSCET). *(a)* Thin Hu-Friedy EL3C elevator. *(b and c)* Hu-Friedy Orban knife KO1/2IU. *(d)* Periotome.

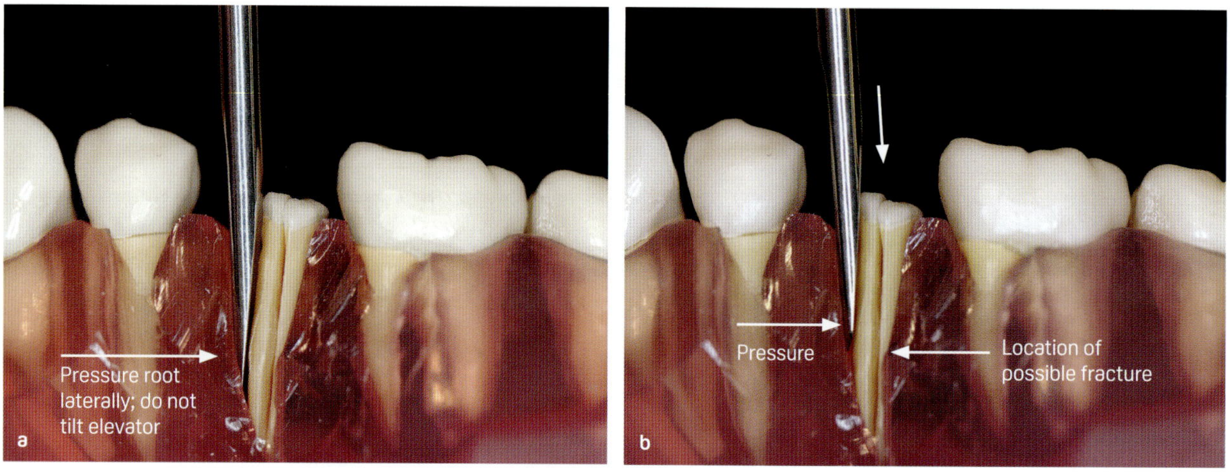

FIG 7-22 *(a)* Placement of the thin elevator as far apically as possible in the periodontal ligament space to pressure, rather than tilt, the root. *(b)* If the thin elevator is positioned only halfway down the root surface, there is a greater chance the root will fracture as it is pressured into the space created by sectioning the root. Pressure on the coronal half of the sectioned root stresses the mid-root area, leading to possible fracture, even if it is fully sectioned through the apex.

Enter Sulcus Laterally and Pressure Roots into Sectioned Space

Using an Orban knife, periotome, or thin elevator, enter the sulcus on the mesial and distal surfaces of the roots and attempt to force the root halves into the space created by sectioning the root (Fig 7-21). It is important to make sure the instrument is seated as far apically as possible into the sulcus so the root is pressured laterally rather than tilted, which may cause the root tip to fracture (Fig 7-22).

Be aware that you are pressuring against the adjacent bone, so do this in a gentle manner, paying attention to the integrity of the adjacent bone. As before, use thin irrigation and suction tips that reach the apex of the roots you are sectioning to irrigate and suction drill cuts. You may find that reentering the sectioned area and cutting between the root sections again may be required. If this does not mobilize the root fragments, it may be necessary to section the root fragments themselves (see next section).

Once root segments are mobilized, individual pieces can be removed with a hemostat or tweezers. Lock the hemostat or tweezers onto a mobile root segment as far apically as possible and use a gentle back-and-forth motion with constant pulling pressure to remove the root segment from the socket (Fig 7-23). This technique is helpful in many instances in which a tooth fragment has been mobilized and needs to be removed.

After one root section is removed, pressure the remaining root section into the space created by removal of the first (RSCET; Figs 7-24a and 7-24b). Then remove this second root half (Figs 7-24c and 7-24d).

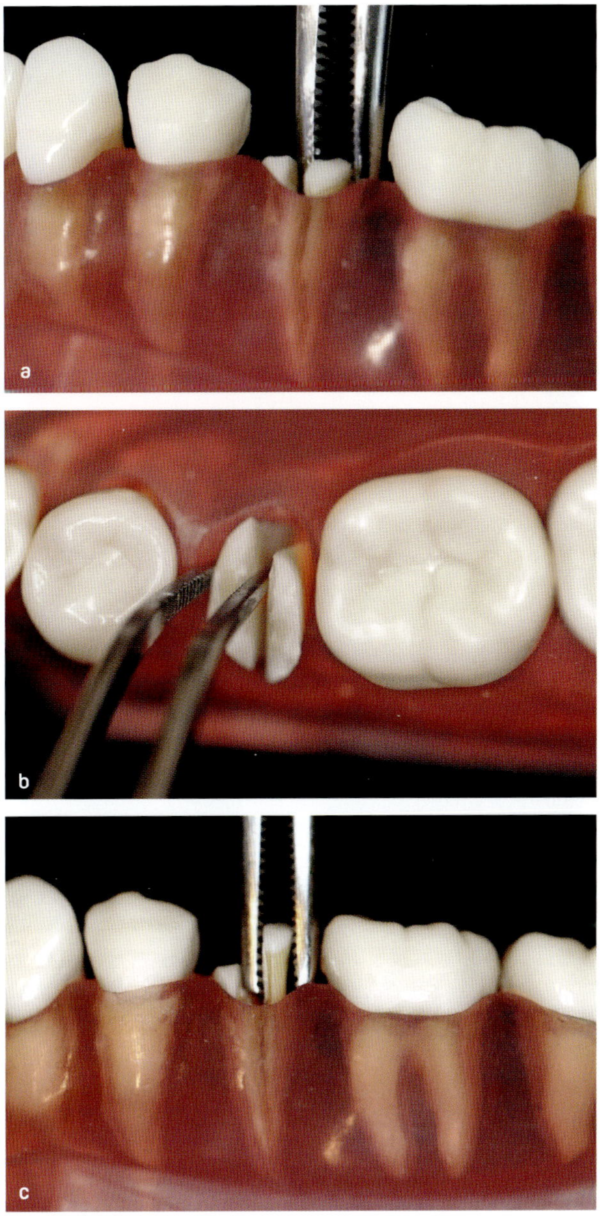

FIG 7-23 *(a)* Hemostat locked onto a mobile root segment. *(b)* Tweezers locked onto a mobile root segment. *(c)* A gentle back-and-forth motion with constant pulling pressure is used to remove the root segment from the socket.

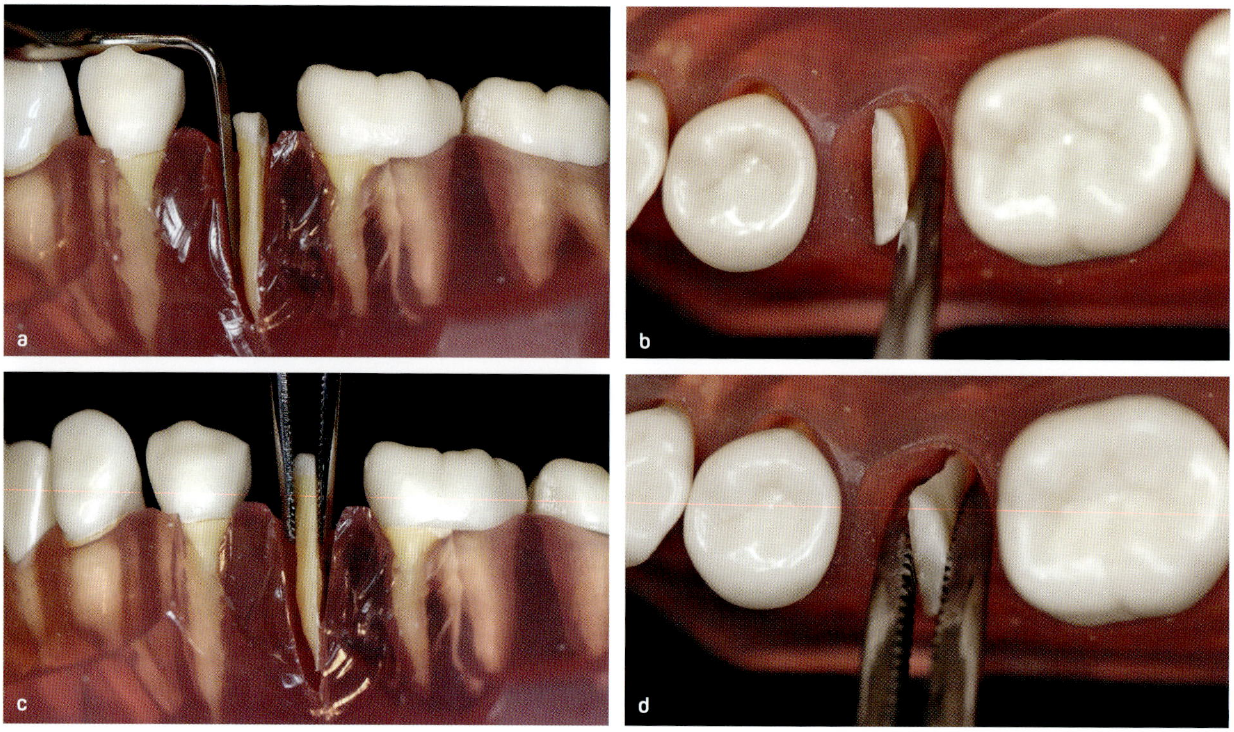

FIG 7-24 *(a and b)* Using a Hu-Friedy Orban knife KO1/2IU to pressure the remaining root section into the space created when the initial half of the root was removed (RSCET). *(c and d)* Once this remaining root half has been mobilized into the root space, it can be removed with a hemostat or tweezers.

Section Roots Again; Pressure into Space Created

If the root halves cannot be mobilized and removed, consider vertically sectioning one and possibly both root halves so they are in quarters, being careful to avoid the mesial and distal socket walls. This is more applicable to larger roots, but smaller roots may require this step, at which time you are actually drilling out most of the root. Again, it is necessary to drill through the apex; feeling the bur drop into softer bone is an indication that you are past the apex. Then, pressure those root quarters into the space created (RSCET) and remove them.

Once root removal is complete, proceed to socket debridement (see chapter 11).

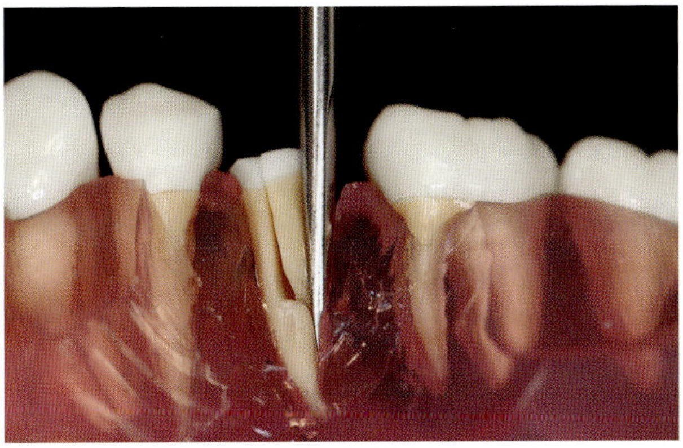

FIG 7-25 If horizontal fracture occurs, the first step is to remove the loose root fragment.

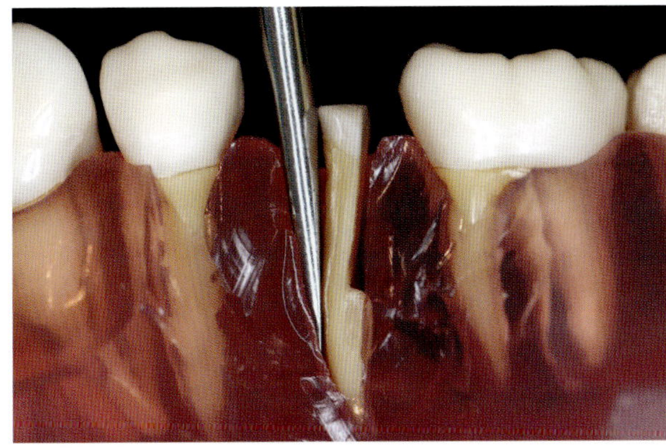

FIG 7-26 The thin Directa Luxator L2S elevator is used to pressure the remaining root, with apex attached, into the space created by removing the root fragment (RSCET).

Complications

If the root is not sectioned entirely through the apex or if the apex fractures, atraumatic removal is difficult. The following steps will help reduce the severity of such complications.

As mentioned earlier, if the root is not sectioned entirely through the apex, pressuring the root into the space may result in a horizontal fracture at the depth of the cut (see Fig 7-19a). If horizontal fracture occurs, remove the loose root fragment (Fig 7-25). The choice is then to attempt to pressure the remaining root, with the apex attached, into the space created by removing the root fragment or to section through the apex.

If the remaining root is pressured into the space created by removing the root fragment (RSCET; Fig 7-26), the risk is another horizontal root fracture, leaving the entire apex. This approach is more successful in softer maxillary bone. Attempting this in the denser mandibular bone will result in fractures more frequently. The other option is to section through the apex (Fig 7-27).

A fractured apex is a complication we will all experience. Sectioning entirely through the apex is necessary to help prevent these complications.

Once root removal is complete, proceed to socket debridement (see chapter 11).

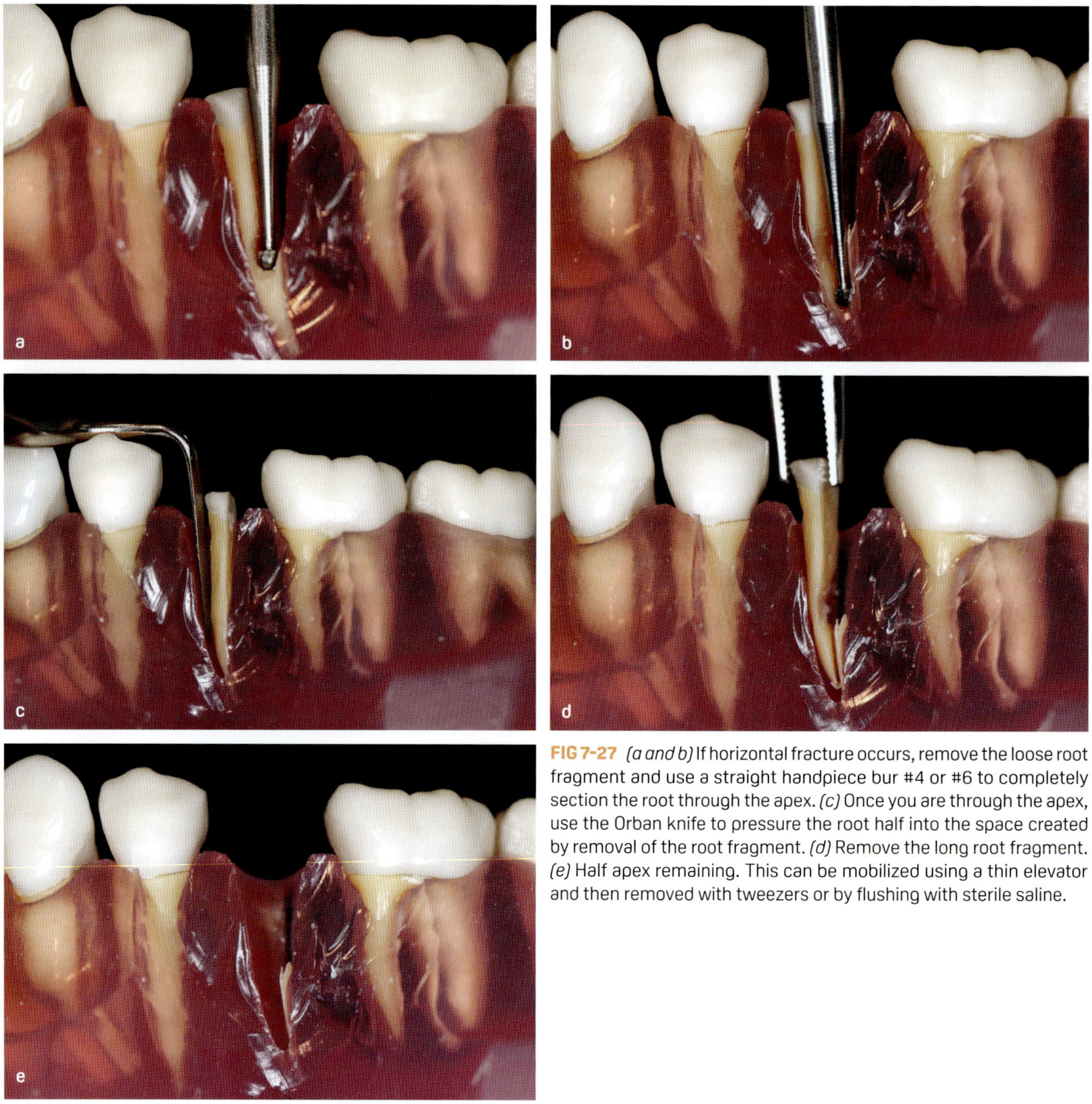

FIG 7-27 *(a and b)* If horizontal fracture occurs, remove the loose root fragment and use a straight handpiece bur #4 or #6 to completely section the root through the apex. *(c)* Once you are through the apex, use the Orban knife to pressure the root half into the space created by removal of the root fragment. *(d)* Remove the long root fragment. *(e)* Half apex remaining. This can be mobilized using a thin elevator and then removed with tweezers or by flushing with sterile saline.

8

Atraumatic Extraction of the Maxillary Premolars: Easy Does It

The following atraumatic extraction techniques apply to maxillary premolars with minimal to no mobility and good bone support. Obviously, teeth with Class II or III mobility can usually be removed atraumatically if there is adequate crown structure to grasp with a forceps. Also, it may not be necessary to use all of the following techniques to atraumatically remove a tooth. Some of the steps may be deemed nonproductive or not applicable to the clinical situation and therefore can be skipped at the discretion of the operating dentist.

Both the maxillary right first and second premolars are used as demonstration examples in this chapter since these teeth have distinctly different root shapes.

Verify Profound Anesthesia

Probe the sulcus with a periodontal probe and stimulate the adjacent gingiva, especially on the palatal, to confirm you have profound anesthesia (Fig 8-1). If anesthesia is inadequate, administer either another nerve block or infiltration into the sulcus and adjacent gingiva circumferentially (Fig 8-2). For quickest onset, use 4% articaine with 1:100,000 epinephrine. For hemostasis, 2% lidocaine 1:100,000 epinephrine is helpful.

A bite block can be used to stabilize the mandible; this also helps patients hold their mouth open during the procedure, reducing muscle fatigue.

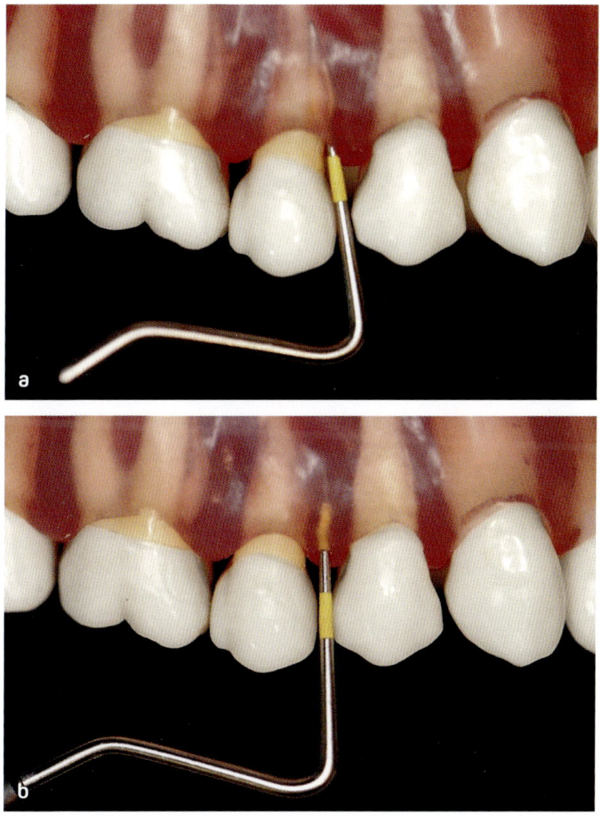

FIG 8-1 Verifying adequate anesthesia. *(a)* Probing the mesiobuccal sulcus of the maxillary right second premolar. *(b)* Probing the gingiva between the maxillary right first and second premolars.

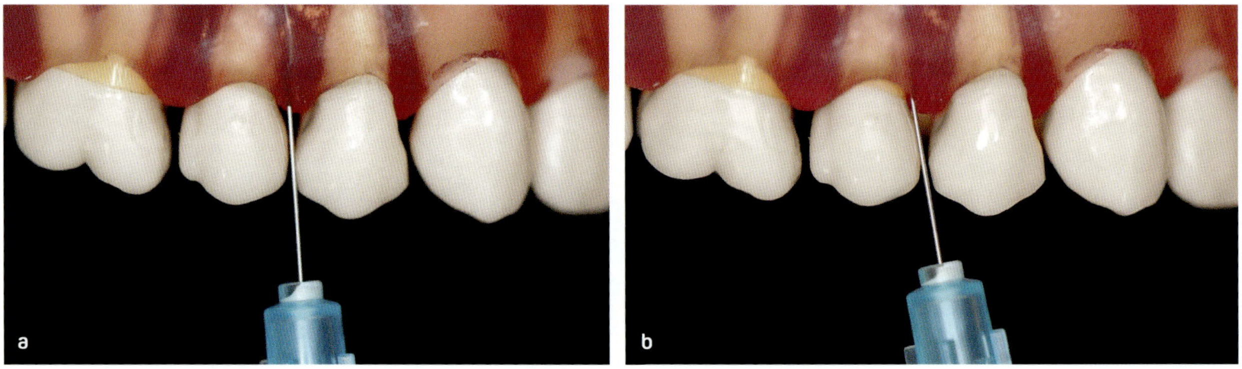

FIG 8-2 Supplementing anesthesia in adjacent gingiva and sulcus. *(a)* Infiltration into the papilla between the maxillary right first and second premolars. *(b)* Infiltration into the mesiobuccal sulcus of the maxillary right second premolar.

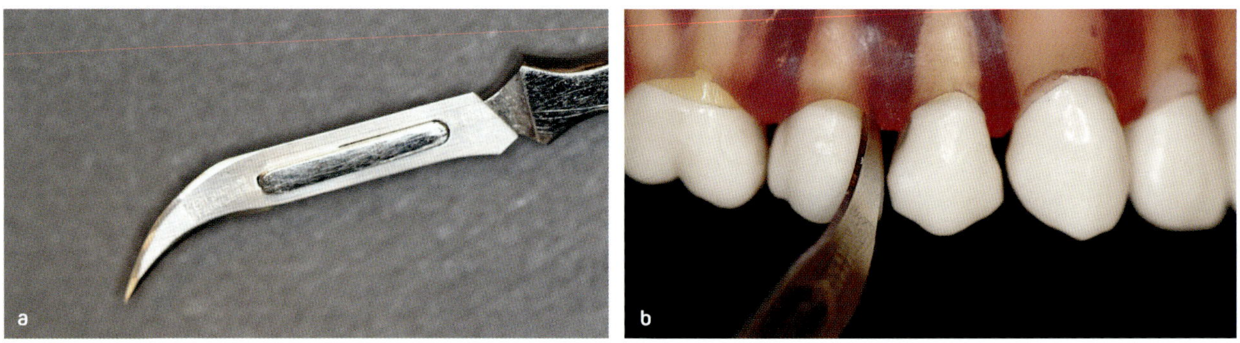

FIG 8-3 *(a)* A 12D scalpel blade. *(b)* The scalpel blade inserted into the mesiobuccal sulcus of the maxillary right second premolar to release the periodontal ligament fibers using a back-and-forth rocking motion with vertical pressure.

Release Periodontal Ligament Fibers Without Flap Reflection

Note that some practitioners remove the crown as the first step. They feel that getting the crown out of the way and just dealing with the root(s) is the most efficient and atraumatic method to remove a tooth. For the purposes of this chapter, we will assume the crown will be left in place for these initial procedures.

Using a 12D scalpel blade, enter the sulcus on the mesial, distal, and palatal, but not the buccal due to the thin buccal bone being vulnerable to resorption and fracture. Apply vertical pressure with a back-and-forth rocking motion (Fig 8-3).

Optional procedure

Use a periotome to excise the periodontal ligament as deeply as possible two times in the mesial, distal, and palatal sulci (Fig 8-4). Avoid the buccal, where the bone is thin. Use a back-and-forth motion with vertical pressure. However, it may be difficult to get into the periodontal ligament space due to lack of space or ankylosis. If that is the case, proceed to the recommended procedure below.

Recommended procedure

Use a surgical-length ¼ round high-speed bur to further sever the periodontal ligament fibers (Fig 8-5a). Use an up-and-down pumping motion in the periodontal ligament space at the mesial, distal, and palatal, but avoid the buccal since the thin buccal bone is vulnerable to resorption and fracture (Fig 8-5b). Extend as far apically as possible, gently pressuring in the direction of the tooth root rather than the bone of the socket wall. This opening of the periodontal ligament space releases the tooth from the adjacent bone, making it easier to remove, and creates space for a thin elevator to enter and pressure the root.

A periotome, scalpel, or ¼ round high-speed bur can be used in any order.

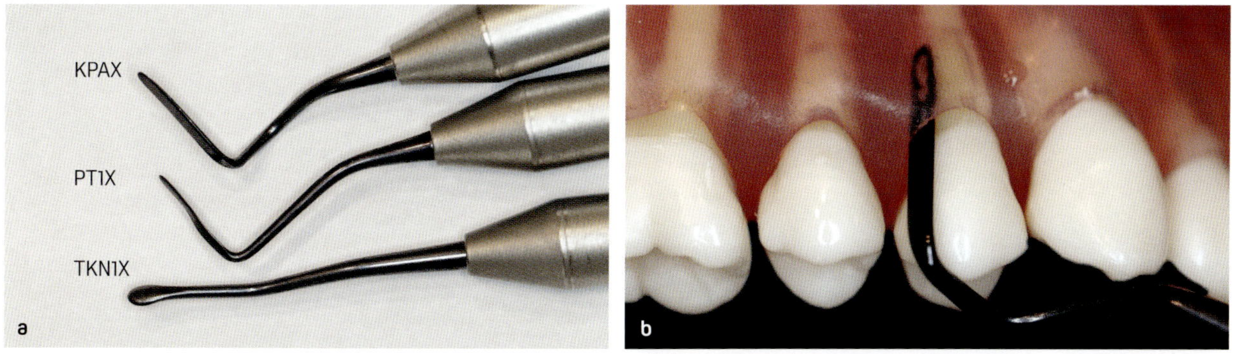

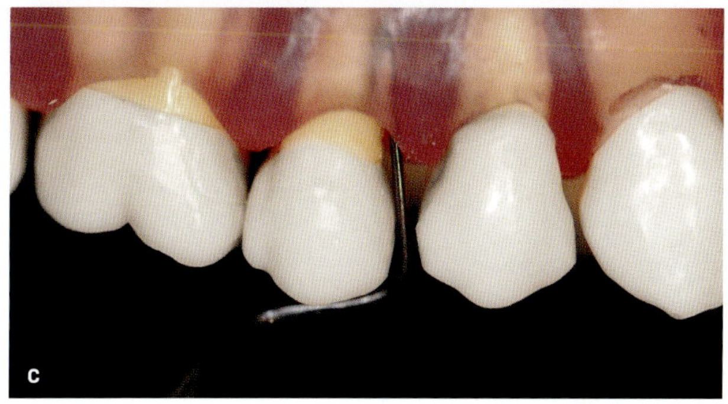

FIG 8-4 *(a)* Hu-Friedy periotomes. *(b)* Periotome inserted into the distobuccal sulcus of the maxillary right first premolar to excise periodontal ligament fibers. Use vertical pressure and a back-and-forth rocking motion. Avoid the thin buccal bone. *(c)* Periotome inserted into the mesial sulcus of the maxillary right second premolar.

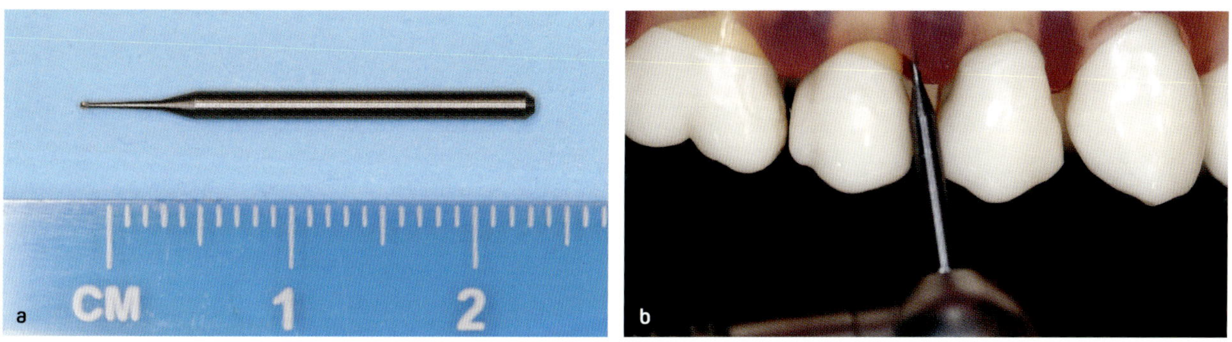

FIG 8-5 *(a)* Surgical-length ¼ round high-speed bur used to separate the root from the bone in the sulcus. *(b)* The bur is inserted in the sulcus with an up-and-down pumping motion with light pressure against the root, not the bone.

Attempt Tooth Removal Coronally Without Flap Reflection

Introduce a thin elevator (Fig 8-6) at the mesiobuccal and distobuccal and, using a twisting motion, attempt to move the tooth coronally (Fig 8-7).

At this point, if the tooth cannot be mobilized with a thin elevator or if there is not enough crown present to luxate the tooth but the root is intact, you can use the Easy X-Trac System (A. Titan) or Benex Root Extraction System (Meisinger) (see chapter 12). Both of these systems involve drilling a hole down the middle of the root canal space and inserting a threaded rod. This rod is pulled coronally with a wedging device, removing the root in one piece. To accomplish this, the crown must be cut horizontally approximately 1 mm above the gingival margin, being aware of the gingival margin location to avoid lacerating the gingiva. Since the roots are tapered, there is minimal trauma when they are removed in a vertical direction with the Easy X-Trac or Benex. In my opinion, this is the most atraumatic method of removing a single-rooted tooth with a tapered root. This will probably apply more often to maxillary second premolars since their roots are wider

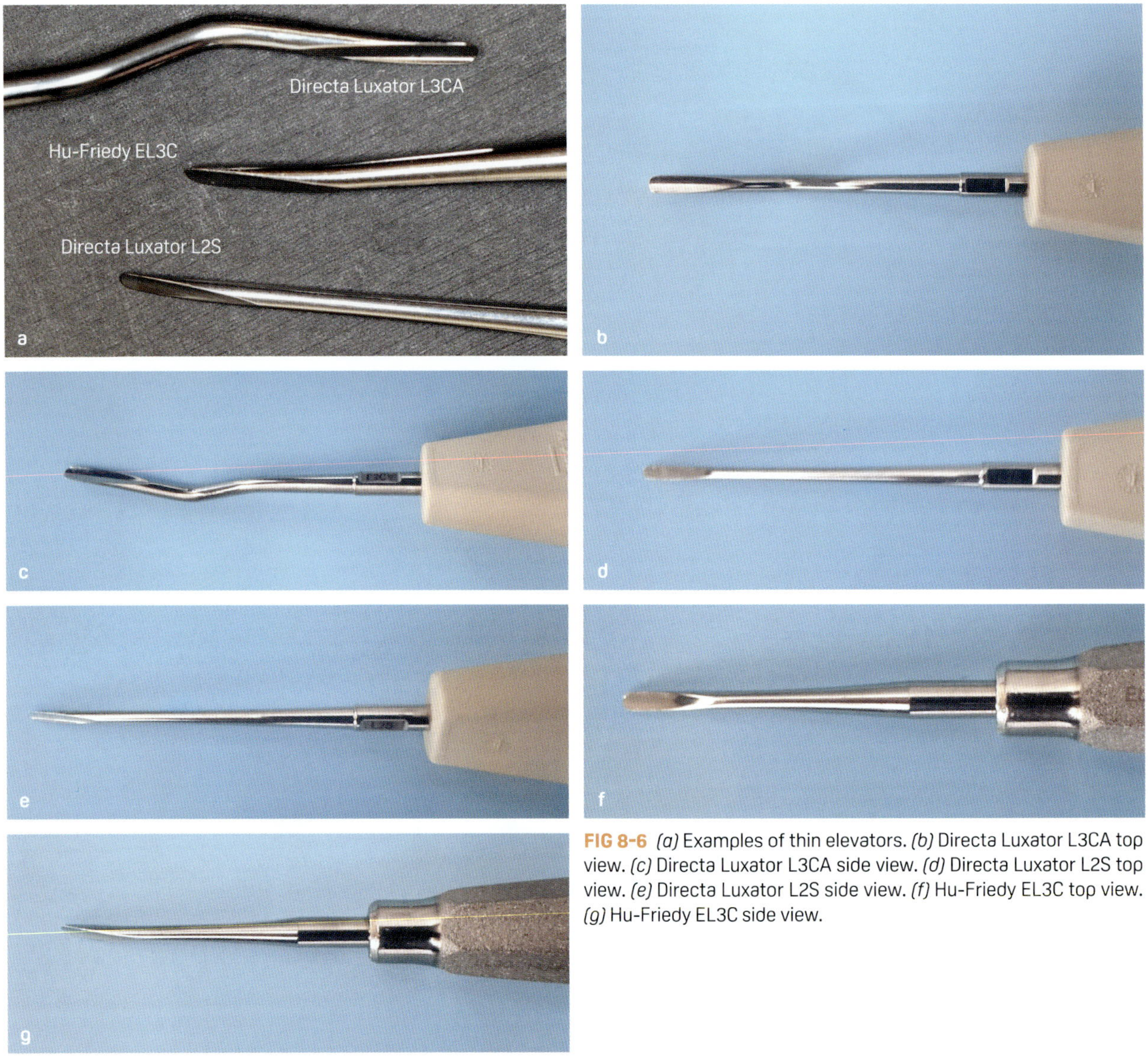

FIG 8-6 *(a)* Examples of thin elevators. *(b)* Directa Luxator L3CA top view. *(c)* Directa Luxator L3CA side view. *(d)* Directa Luxator L2S top view. *(e)* Directa Luxator L2S side view. *(f)* Hu-Friedy EL3C top view. *(g)* Hu-Friedy EL3C side view.

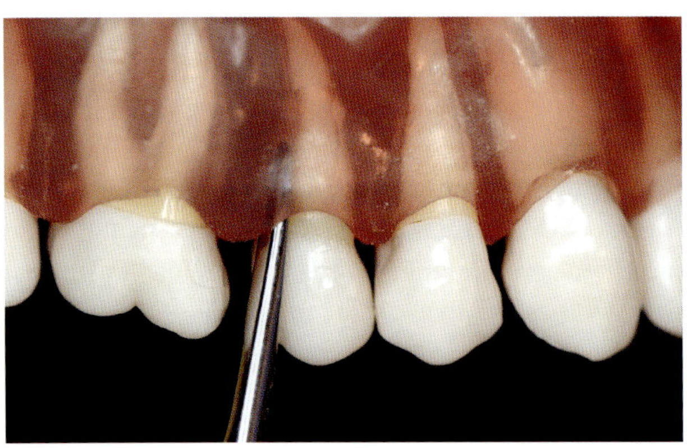

FIG 8-7 Thin Directa Luxator L2S elevator inserted at the distobuccal of the maxillary right second premolar.

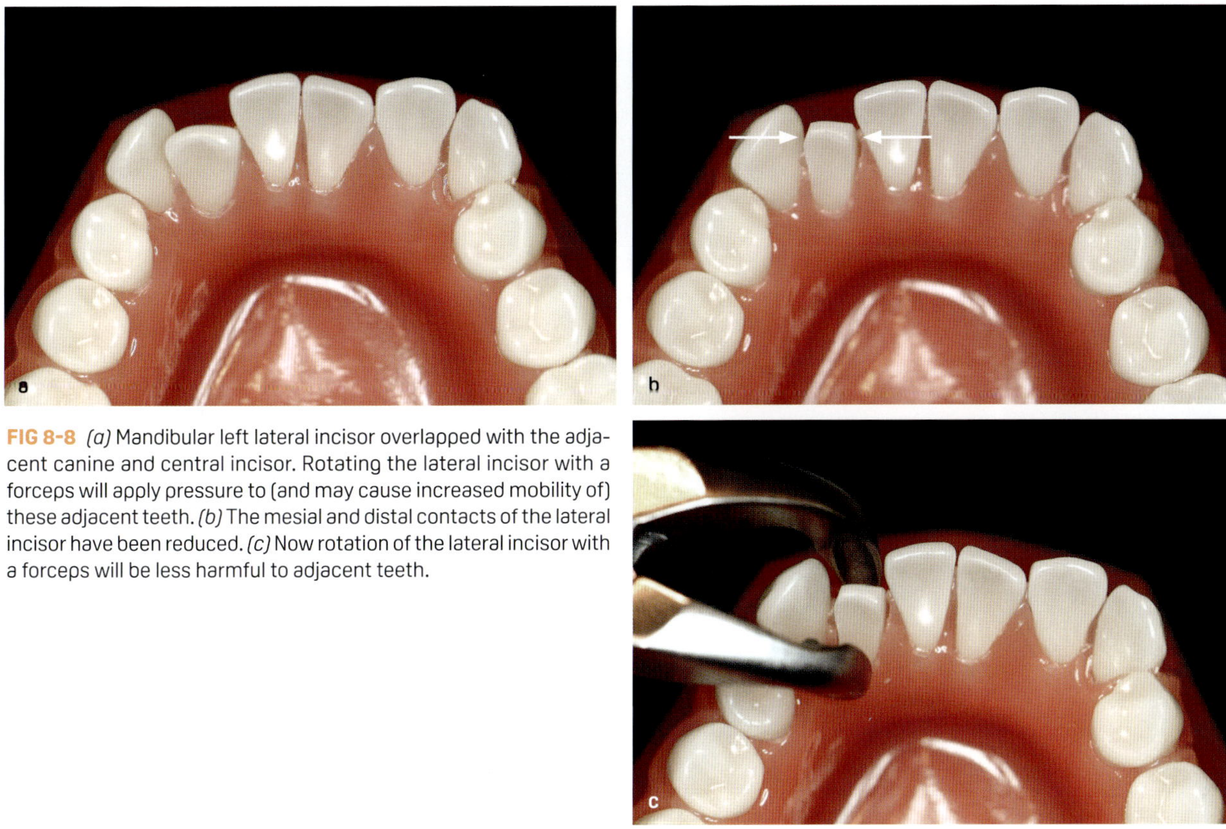

FIG 8-8 *(a)* Mandibular left lateral incisor overlapped with the adjacent canine and central incisor. Rotating the lateral incisor with a forceps will apply pressure to (and may cause increased mobility of) these adjacent teeth. *(b)* The mesial and distal contacts of the lateral incisor have been reduced. *(c)* Now rotation of the lateral incisor with a forceps will be less harmful to adjacent teeth.

and generally more often fused than those of the maxillary first premolars. With the latter, you will need to decide which root—buccal or palatal—has enough room to allow a threaded rod to be inserted with sufficient retention to remove the root.

However, if there is adequate crown structure present for luxation of any kind, the following may be helpful.

Reduce Interproximal Contacts

We are attempting to remove a tooth as atraumatically as possible, and this pertains not only to the tooth being extracted but also to the adjacent teeth, their restorations, and the rest of the mouth as well. If we were to rotate a tooth with tight or overlapping contacts, we would be pressuring the adjacent contacts and therefore moving the adjacent teeth. (If multiple adjacent teeth are being removed, this concept does not apply; luxation of a tooth with tight or overlapping contacts may actually help loosen adjacent teeth planned for extraction.) Therefore, where teeth are overlapped or crowded, I feel it is important to reduce the interproximal contacts on a single tooth to be removed. Note that if interproximal contacts are present, but luxation does not move or harm adjacent teeth or restorations, then reduction of interproximal contacts is not necessary. If contacts are overlapping on one side only, rotate the tooth in the direction that does not increase contact pressure. Figure 8-8 presents overlapping mandibular incisors as an example.

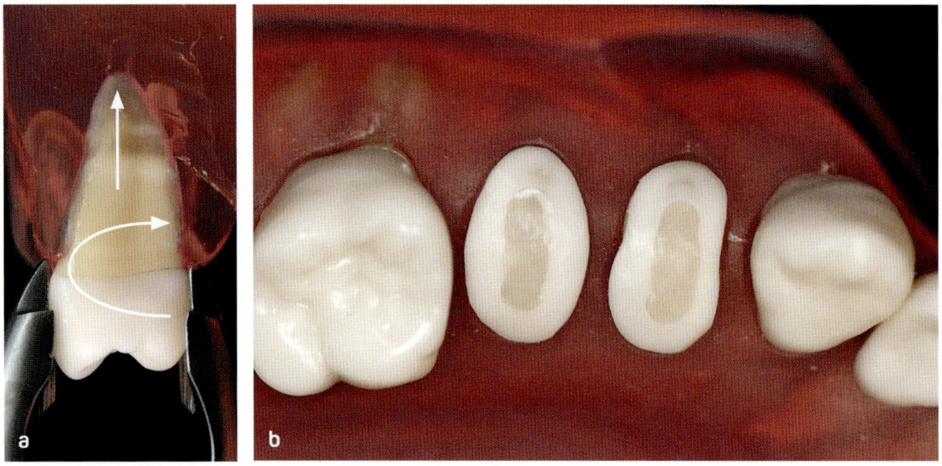

FIG 8-9 *(a)* Forceps applied as far apically as possible without damaging bone or soft tissue. First apply vertical pressure, then rotational movement. *(b)* Crowns removed to show root anatomy. The maxillary right second premolar root is oval shaped, while the first premolar root is shaped like a figure eight. Excessive rotation of either may fracture the socket wall or root.

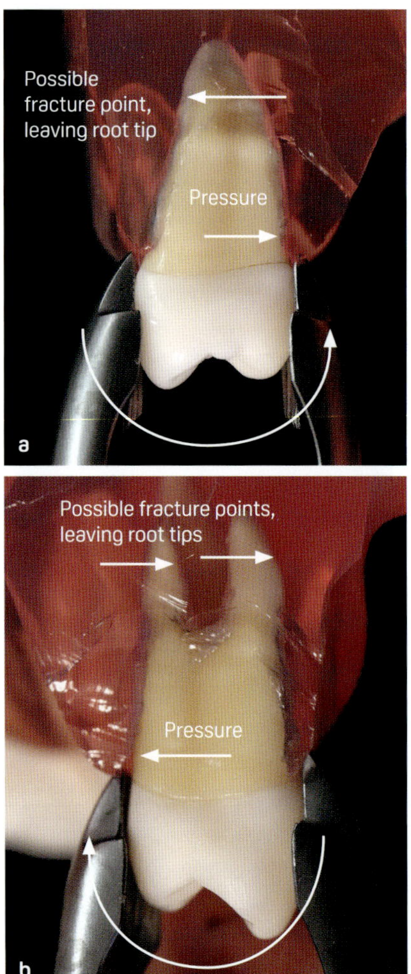

FIG 8-10 Pressure applied coronally toward the palatal of the maxillary right second *(a)* and first *(b)* premolars, which also pressures the buccal surface of the roots. This may result in fracture of the apices.

Luxate Gently with Forceps

To gently luxate the tooth, place forceps as far apically as possible without engaging bone. Try to engage the root surface apical to any restoration margins. Gently apply pressure apically and hold for 30 seconds. While continuing to apply apical pressure, gently luxate in a buccal and palatal direction with slight rotation to test the mobility of the tooth (Fig 8-9a). The reason for applying apical pressure while luxating is that it shifts the axis of rotation in an apical direction, reducing the chance for root fracture. Remember, the maxillary first premolar roots are shaped like a figure eight, and the maxillary second premolar roots are oval in shape (Fig 8-9b). It is recommended to avoid excessive rotation of either since that would expand the socket and could fracture the socket wall or the root.

If the bone on the buccal or palatal alveolar crest is especially thick, pressure can be placed in that respective direction. However, it is important to realize that when applying pressure coronally in a lateral direction toward the alveolar crest, the apical portion of the tooth will be forced against the opposite socket wall. This pressure can lead to fracture of the apex, leaving a root tip to retrieve. Mandibular bone is denser than maxillary bone; therefore, root fracture is more probable in the mandible, depending on the root anatomy. Maxillary first premolar roots are bifurcated, and the apices can fracture easily; maxillary second premolars generally have fused roots, but the apices are still vulnerable to fracture (Fig 8-10).

If there is a full-coverage restoration, luxation may or may not remove the crown. If gentle luxation is not successful in removing the tooth, the crown (whether a cemented full-coverage restoration or natural tooth) should be sectioned horizontally about 1 mm coronal to the gingival margin as described in the next section.

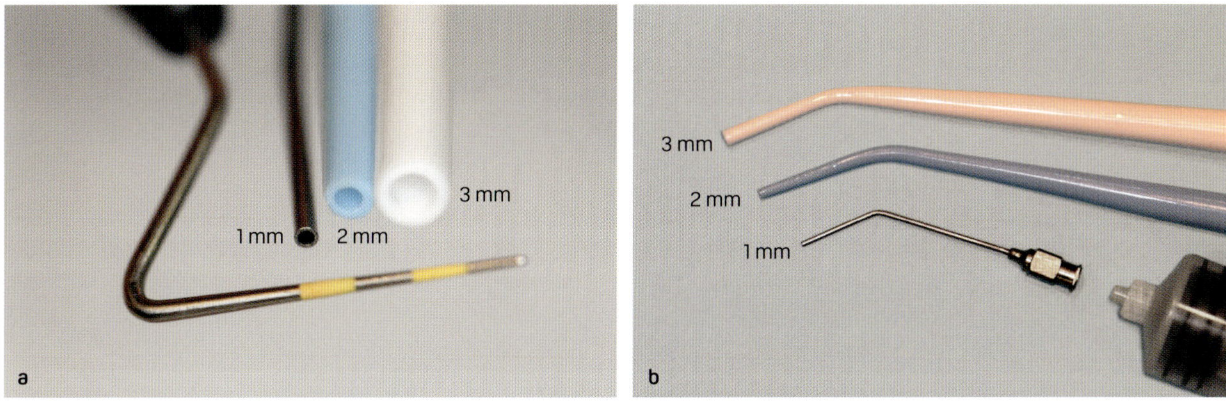

FIG 8-11 *(a and b)* Thin 1-mm irrigation tip and 2- and 3-mm-diameter suction tips used during sectioning of a crown.

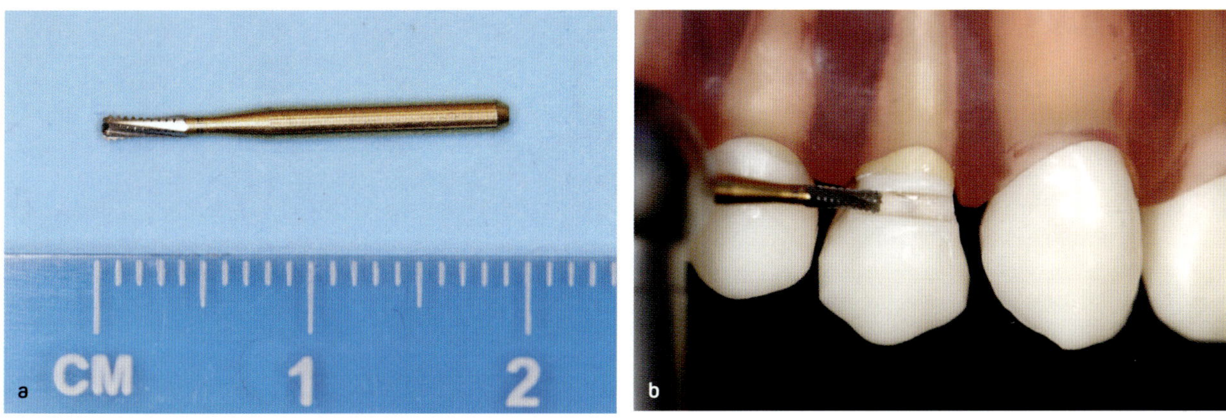

FIG 8-12 *(a)* Great White high-speed crosscut fissure bur used to horizontally section the crown. *(b)* Sectioning the maxillary right first premolar 1 mm coronal to the free gingival margin.

Section Crown Horizontally at the Cementoenamel Junction

Some practitioners go right to this step for every extraction, feeling that it is the most efficient and atraumatic method.

When sectioning a crown or roots, it is important to use plenty of saline irrigation with a thin irrigation tip to remove tooth debris and to use thin suction tips to suction within the drill cuts (Fig 8-11). This allows you to see and feel in these areas. Section the crown 1 mm coronal to the gingival margin using a Great White (SS White) high-speed crosscut fissure bur (Fig 8-12). It is important to be aware of the gingival margin location to avoid lacerating the gingiva.

Obviously, it's much easier to section through tooth structure or a composite restoration as compared to a metal restoration. Regardless of the material, section two-thirds of the way through the crown, and then, using an elevator, gently pry off the crown. Using a football-shaped high-speed diamond bur, smooth the remaining tooth structure to a fairly flat surface approximately 1 mm coronal to the gingival margin (Fig 8-13).

Removing the crown allows you to see the remaining root structure anatomy and determine the best location to section vertically. Vertical fractures may be evident also. A dye such as To Dye For (Roydent) may be used to help visualize possible fractures.

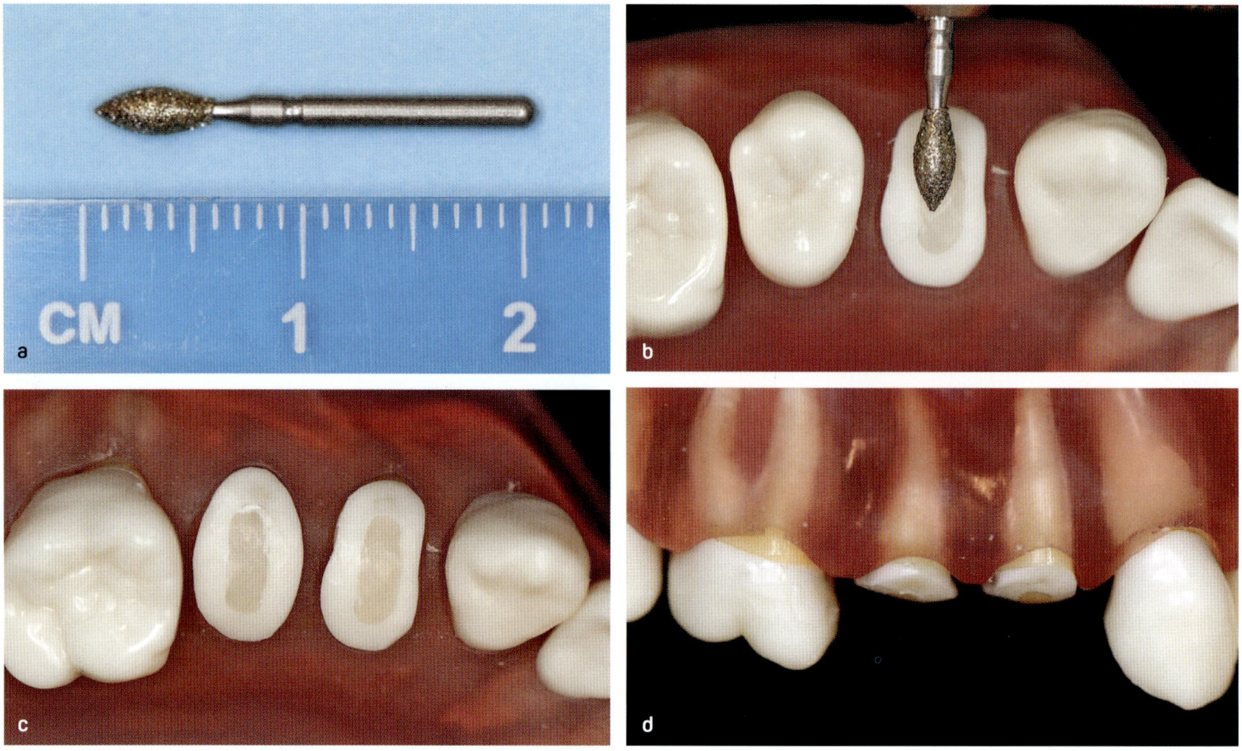

FIG 8-13 *(a)* High-speed football diamond bur used to smooth the remaining root to a level 1 mm above the gingival margin after sectioning off the crown. *(b)* Bur used to smooth the remaining root of the maxillary right first premolar. *(c and d)* Occlusal and buccal views of the maxillary right premolars sectioned horizontally 1 mm above the gingival margin.

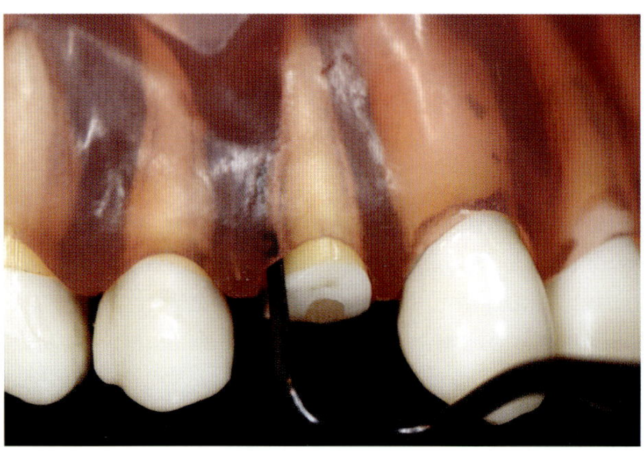

FIG 8-14 Periotome in the distal sulcus of the maxillary right first premolar using vertical pressure and a back-and-forth rocking motion. Avoid the buccal, where bone is thin.

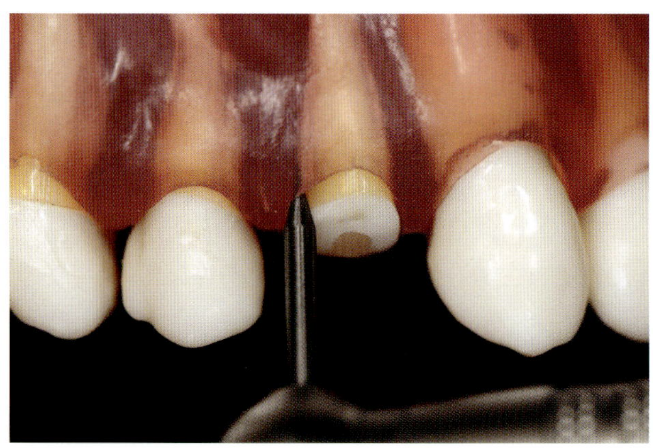

FIG 8-15 Surgical-length ¼ round high-speed bur used with a gentle up-and-down motion in the sulcus, exerting pressure toward the root, not the bone of the socket wall.

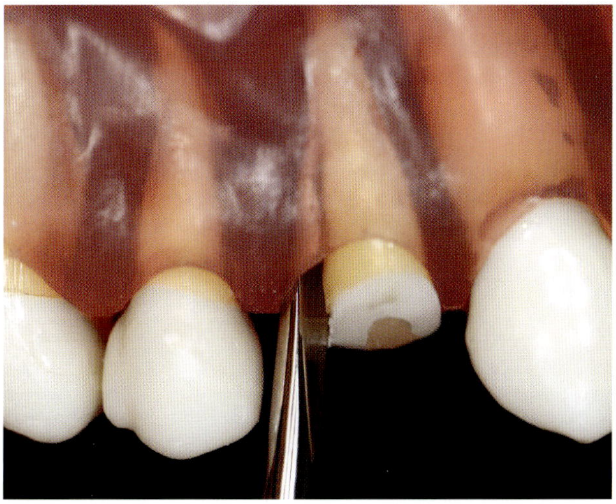

FIG 8-16 A thin Hu-Friedy EL3C elevator is used to gently luxate the root with a twisting motion, attempting to elevate it out of the socket.

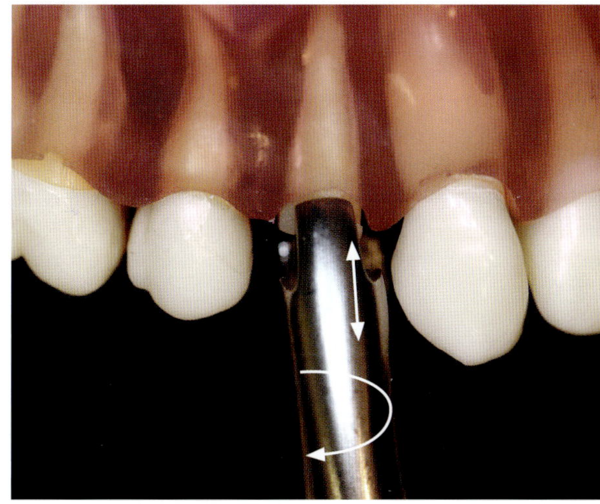

FIG 8-17 Using forceps to mobilize the maxillary right first premolar root.

Optional procedure

Release the periodontal ligament fibers again using a narrow periotome (see Fig 8-4a). Enter the sulcus on the palatal, mesial, and distal, applying vertical pressure and a back-and-forth rocking motion to excise the periodontal ligament fibers further apically (Fig 8-14).

Recommended procedure

Instead of a periotome, you can use a surgical-length ¼ round high-speed bur to further sever the periodontal ligament fibers (Fig 8-15). Attempt to cut more in the direction of the root rather than the bone of the socket wall. Excising periodontal ligament fibers like this detaches the root from bone, allowing for easier extraction. Avoid the buccal aspect because bone in this area is thin.

Use Thin Elevator to Attempt Root Removal Coronally Without Flap Reflection

Introducing a thin elevator (see Fig 8-6a) at the mesiobuccal and distobuccal, use a twisting motion to attempt to move the root coronally (Fig 8-16). If the root moves but not coronally, release the periodontal ligament fibers again with the periotome or high-speed ¼ round bur, then try the elevators again at the mesiobuccal and distobuccal. If you are not able to remove the root at this point, the next step is to insert the beaks of an incisor forceps as apically as possible and attempt luxation and slight rotation one more time (Fig 8-17).

If this is not successful, the next step is to vertically section the root.

Section Roots Vertically

This technique is termed the *root space creation extraction technique* (*RSCET*). The concept involves using a surgical-length high-speed crosscut fissure bur to remove tooth structure and creating a space into which the root can be pressured, away from the sulcus and socket wall (Fig 8-18a). In this way, a tooth can be removed without removing supporting bone. Single-rooted teeth, like the maxillary second premolars, are usually sectioned in a buccopalatal direction so that mobilization of the root fragments does not stress the buccal bone, but care must be taken to not score the buccal bone (Figs 8-18b and 8-18c). Multirooted teeth, such as the maxillary first premolars, are sectioned mesiodistally between the roots, essentially making them individual roots (Figs 8-18d and 8-18e). This allows them each to be luxated in their own direction, making their removal more atraumatic. It is important that you have thin sterile saline irrigation and suction tips that reach the apices of the roots you are sectioning, allowing you to irrigate and suction the drill cuts, removing tooth debris for visualization.

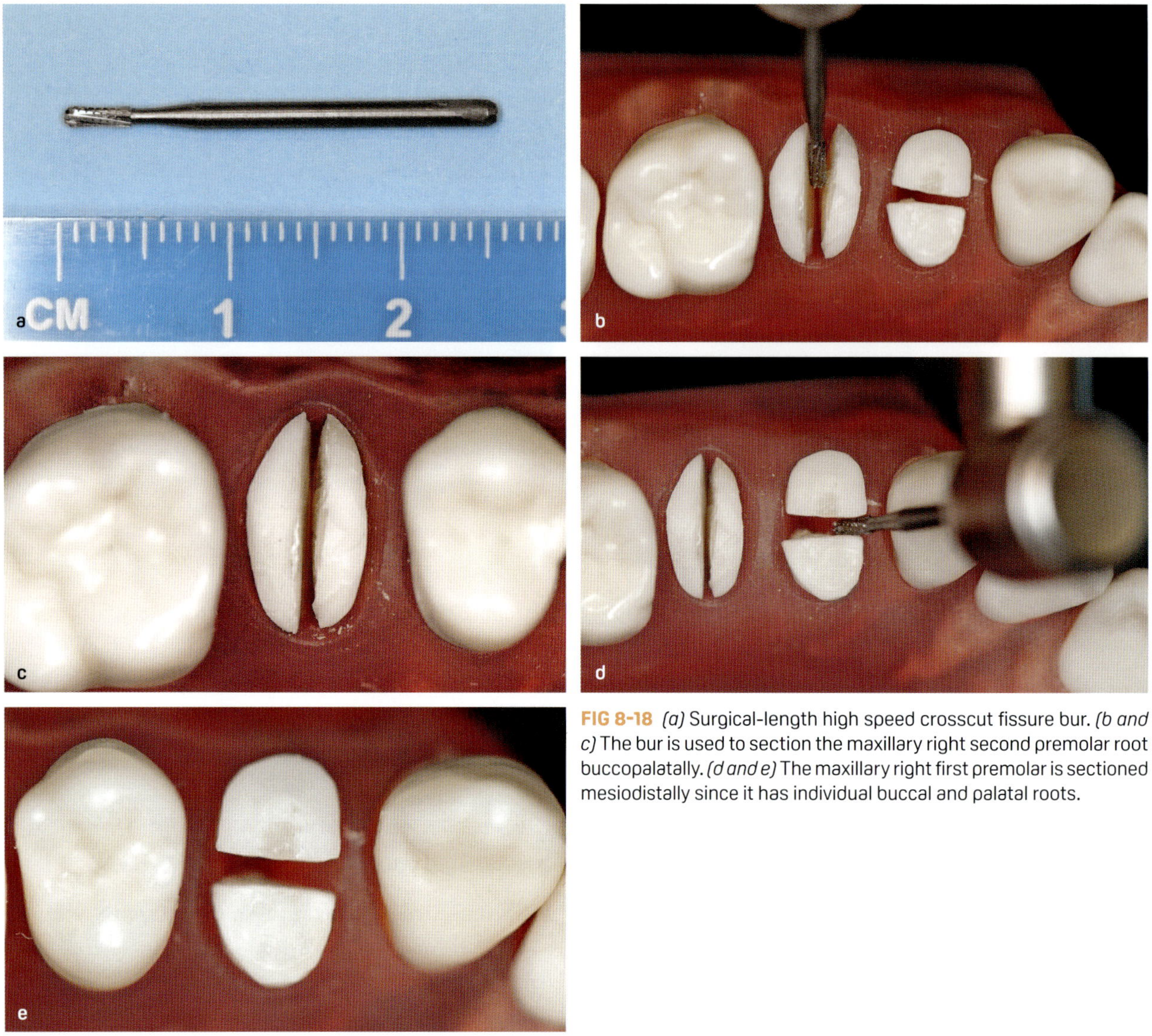

FIG 8-18 *(a)* Surgical-length high speed crosscut fissure bur. *(b and c)* The bur is used to section the maxillary right second premolar root buccopalatally. *(d and e)* The maxillary right first premolar is sectioned mesiodistally since it has individual buccal and palatal roots.

If the root is not sectioned entirely through the apex, pressuring the root into the space may result in a horizontal fracture at the depth of the cut (Fig 8-19a). Therefore, if the surgical-length high-speed crosscut fissure bur does not reach the apex, use a straight handpiece round bur #4 or #6 to complete cutting through the apex. This requires opening up the cut wider at the coronal aspect to allow room for the shank of the straight handpiece bur (Figs 8-19b and 8-19c). When the root is completely sectioned through the apex, you will feel your handpiece "drop" into the softer bone (Fig 8-19d). Since they have separate roots, maxillary first premolars can be sectioned more quickly than maxillary second premolars. On maxillary second premolars, cut toward the palatal and facial slightly to make sure the cut is entirely through the root structure. Maxillary first premolars require a mesiodistal cut because they have individual buccal and palatal roots.

Once you have confirmed that the root has been completely divided through the apex, proceed as follows.

Elevate Gently Between Sectioned Root Pieces

Enter the sectioned space with a thin elevator and gently pressure the root fragments laterally using a twisting motion (Fig 8-20). Be aware that you are also pressuring the bone laterally, so if it looks like there is a weak area, avoid pressuring that area.

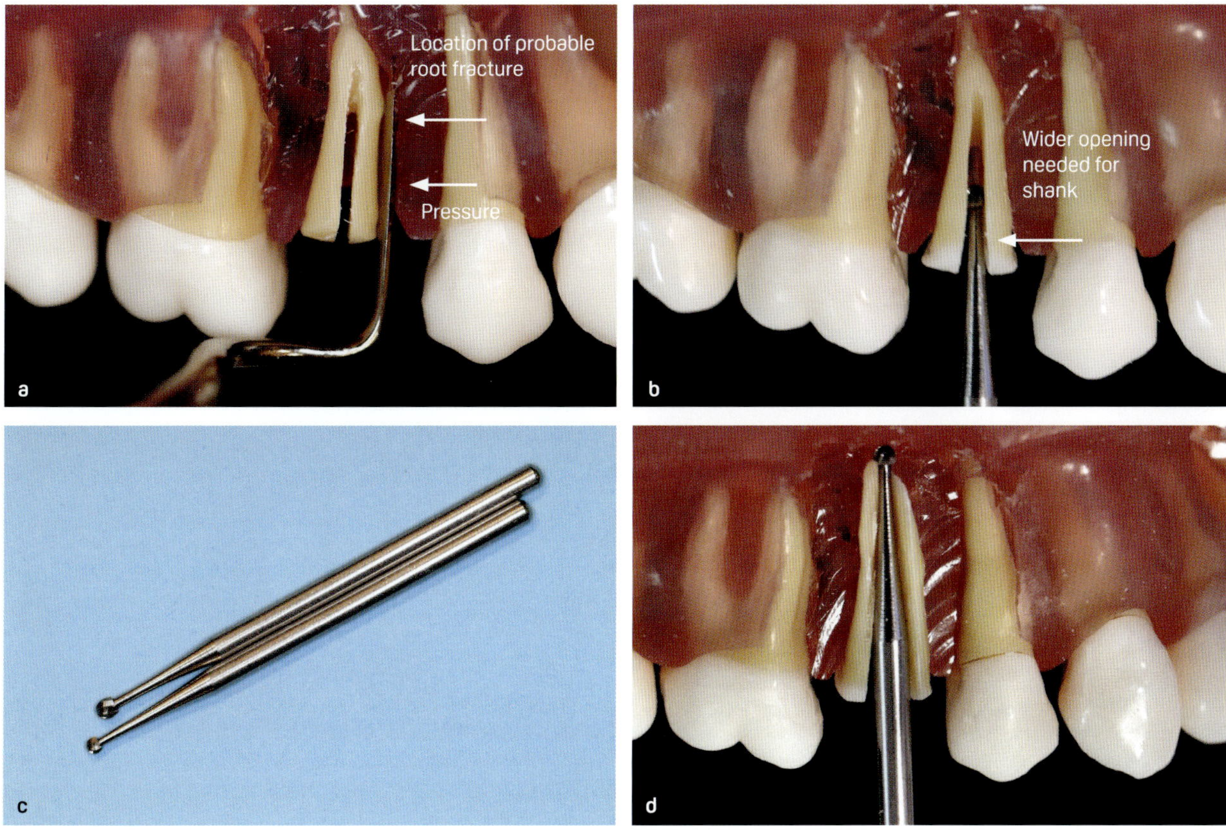

FIG 8-19 *(a)* Orban knife at the mesial of the maxillary right second premolar, pressuring the incompletely sectioned root. There is a risk of fracturing the root at the depth of the cut, leaving the apex attached to the remaining root (gingiva removed for visualization purposes). *(b)* Root not sectioned entirely through apex. A wider opening is needed to allow room for the shank of the straight handpiece bur. *(c)* Straight handpiece burs #6 *(top)* and #4 *(bottom)*; the smaller bur (#4) is used for smaller roots, and #6 is used for larger roots. *(d)* Straight handpiece bur #6 sectioning completely past the apex of the maxillary right second premolar root into bone.

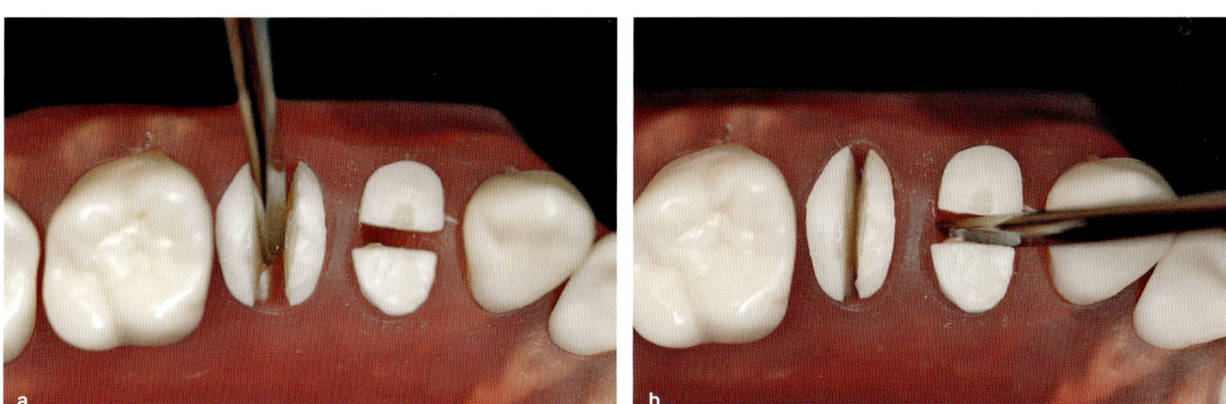

FIG 8-20 Thin Directa Luxator L2S elevator used with a gentle twisting motion to pressure the maxillary right second *(a)* and first *(b)* premolar root sections laterally.

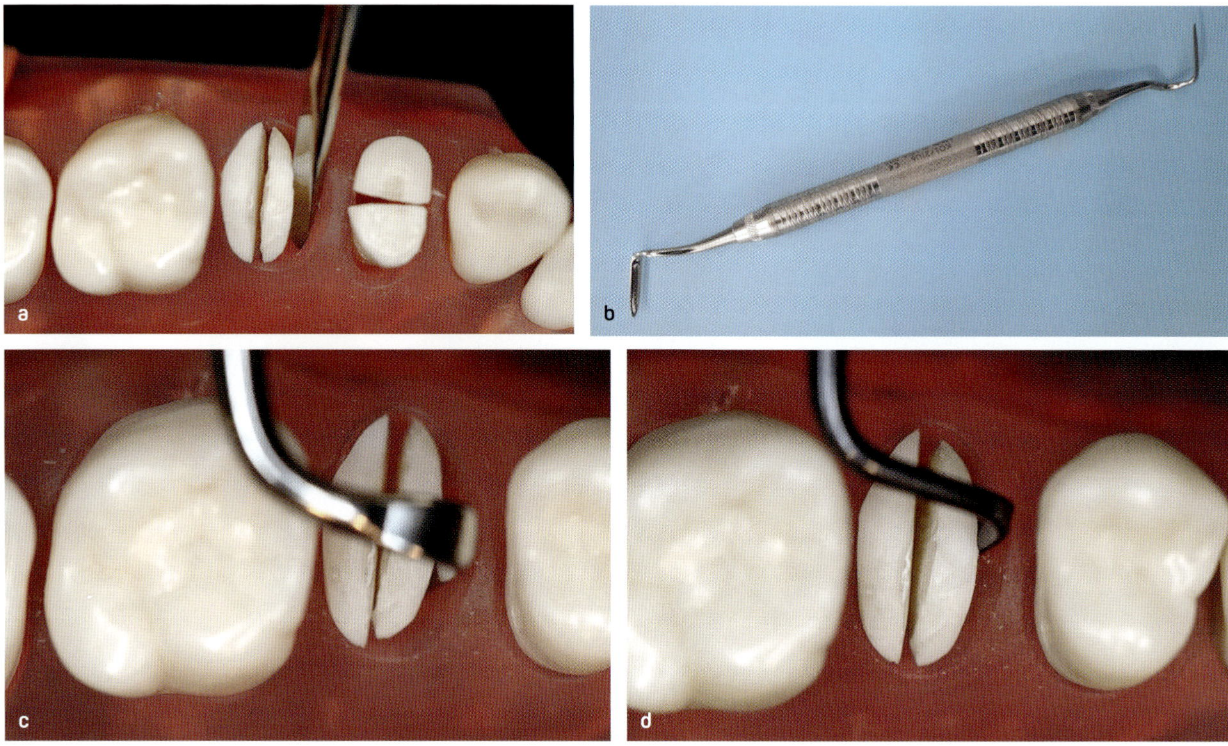

FIG 8-21 Various instruments used with vertical pressure and a back-and-forth rocking motion to pressure the mesial root section of the maxillary right second premolar into the space created by sectioning (RSCET). *(a)* Thin Hu-Friedy EL3C elevator. *(b and c)* Hu-Friedy Orban knife KO1/2IU. *(d)* Periotome.

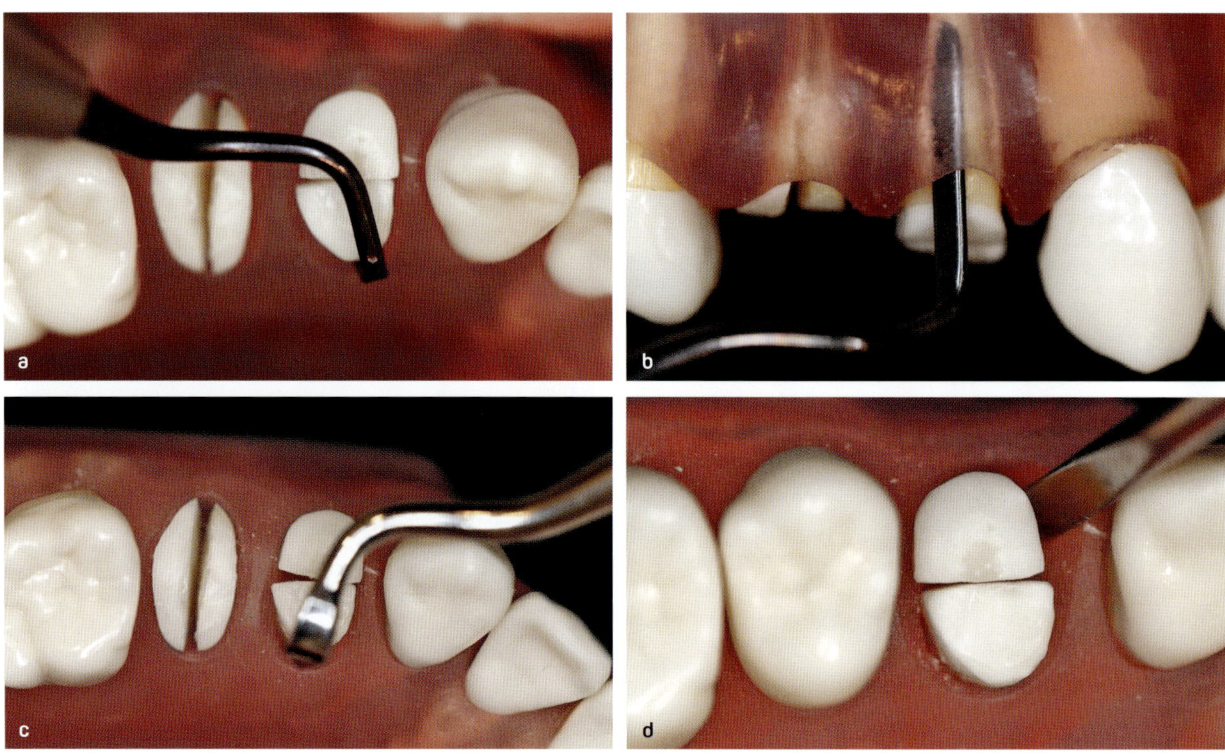

FIG 8-22 Various instruments used with vertical pressure and a back-and-forth rocking motion to pressure the buccal and palatal roots of the maxillary right first premolar into the space created by separating the roots (RSCET). *(a)* Periotome in palatal sulcus. *(b)* Periotome in the buccal sulcus, used with care in this area of thin bone. *(c)* Hu-Friedy Orban knife KO1/2IU in palatal sulcus. *(d)* Thin Hu-Friedy EL3C elevator in mesiobuccal sulcus.

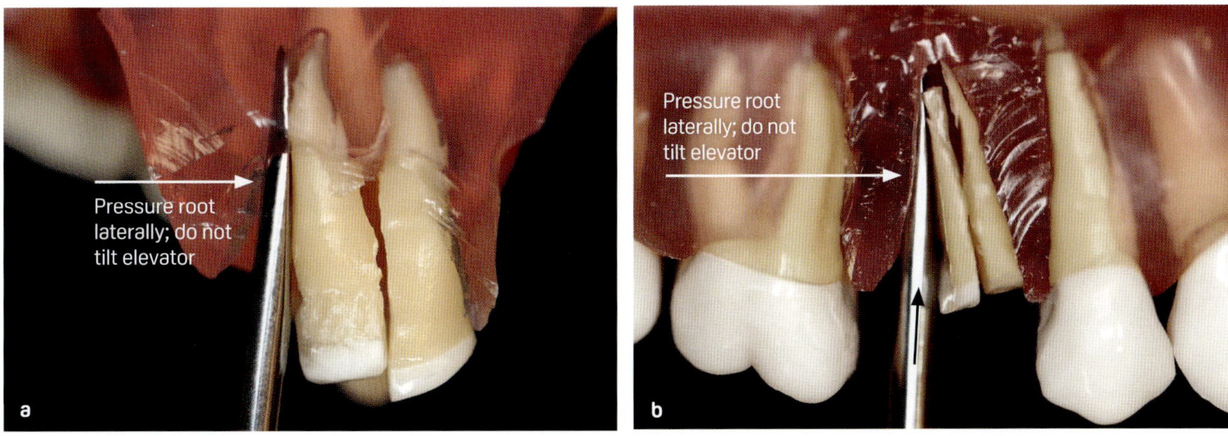

FIG 8-23 Placement of thin Directa Luxator L2S elevator as far apically as possible in the palatal sulcus of the maxillary right first premolar *(a)* and the distal sulcus of the maxillary right second premolar *(b)* to pressure, rather than tilt, the sectioned roots, reducing the risk of root fracture.

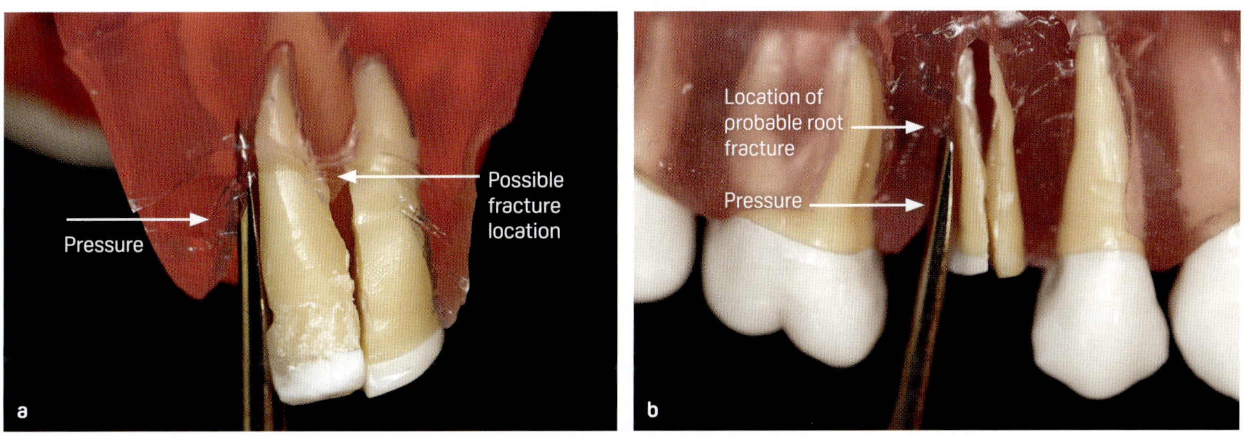

FIG 8-24 *(a and b)* If the thin elevator is positioned only halfway down the root surface, there is a greater chance the root will fracture as it is pressured into the space created by sectioning the roots. Pressure on the coronal half of the sectioned root stresses the mid-root area, leading to possible fracture, even if it is fully sectioned through the apex.

Enter Sulcus Laterally and Pressure Roots into Sectioned Space

Using an Orban knife, periotome, or thin elevator, enter the sulcus and pressure the root halves into the space created by sectioning the roots (Figs 8-21 and 8-22). It is important to make sure the instrument is seated as far apically as possible into the sulcus so the root is pressured laterally rather than tilted, which may cause the root tip to fracture (Figs 8-23 and 8-24).

Be aware that you are pressuring against the adjacent bone, so do this in a gentle manner, paying attention to the integrity of the adjacent bone. As before, use thin irrigation and suction tips that reach the apex of the roots you are sectioning to irrigate and suction drill cuts. You may find that reentering the cut area and sectioning between the roots again may be required. If this does not mobilize the root fragments, it may be necessary to section the fragments themselves or, in the case of maxillary first premolars, the individual roots (see next section).

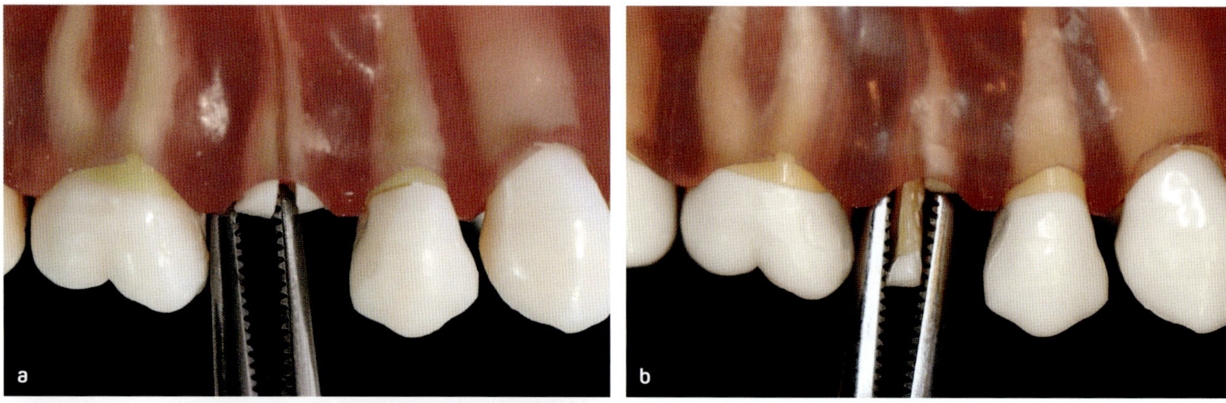

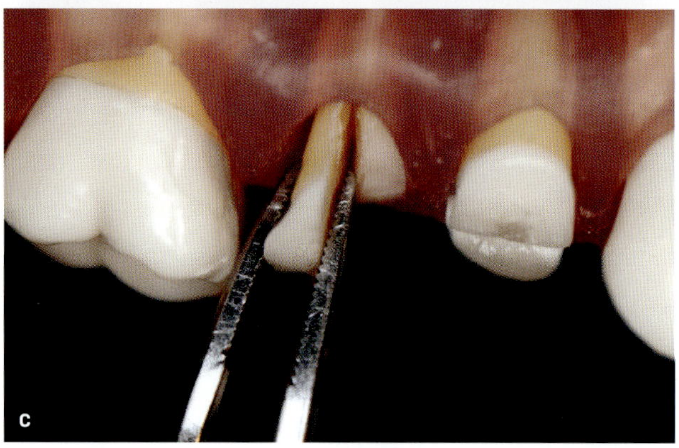

FIG 8-25 *(a)* Hemostat locked onto mobile distal root segment of the maxillary right second premolar. *(b and c)* A gentle back-and-forth motion with constant pulling pressure is used to remove the root segment from the socket.

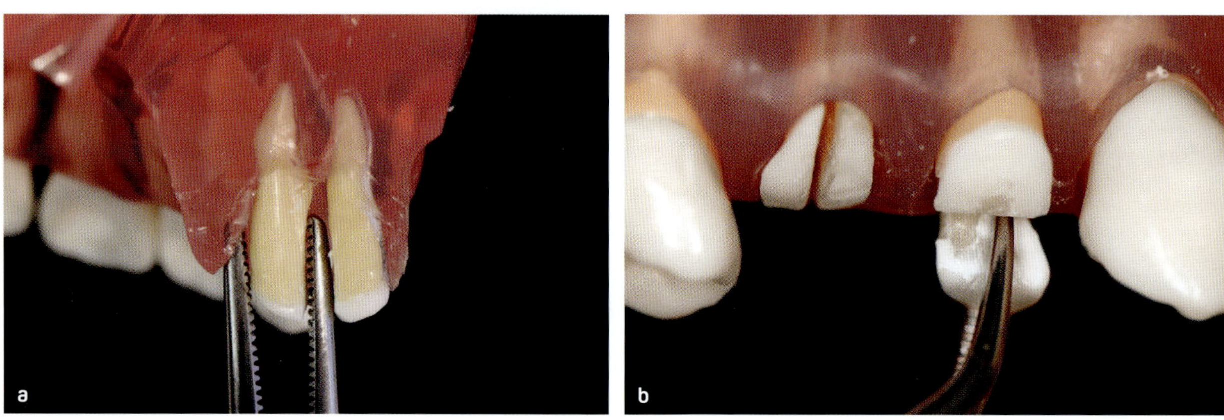

FIG 8-26 *(a)* Hemostat locked as far apically as possible onto the mobile palatal root of the maxillary right first premolar. A gentle back-and-forth motion with constant pulling pressure is used to remove the root segment from the socket. *(b)* Removing the palatal root with tweezers.

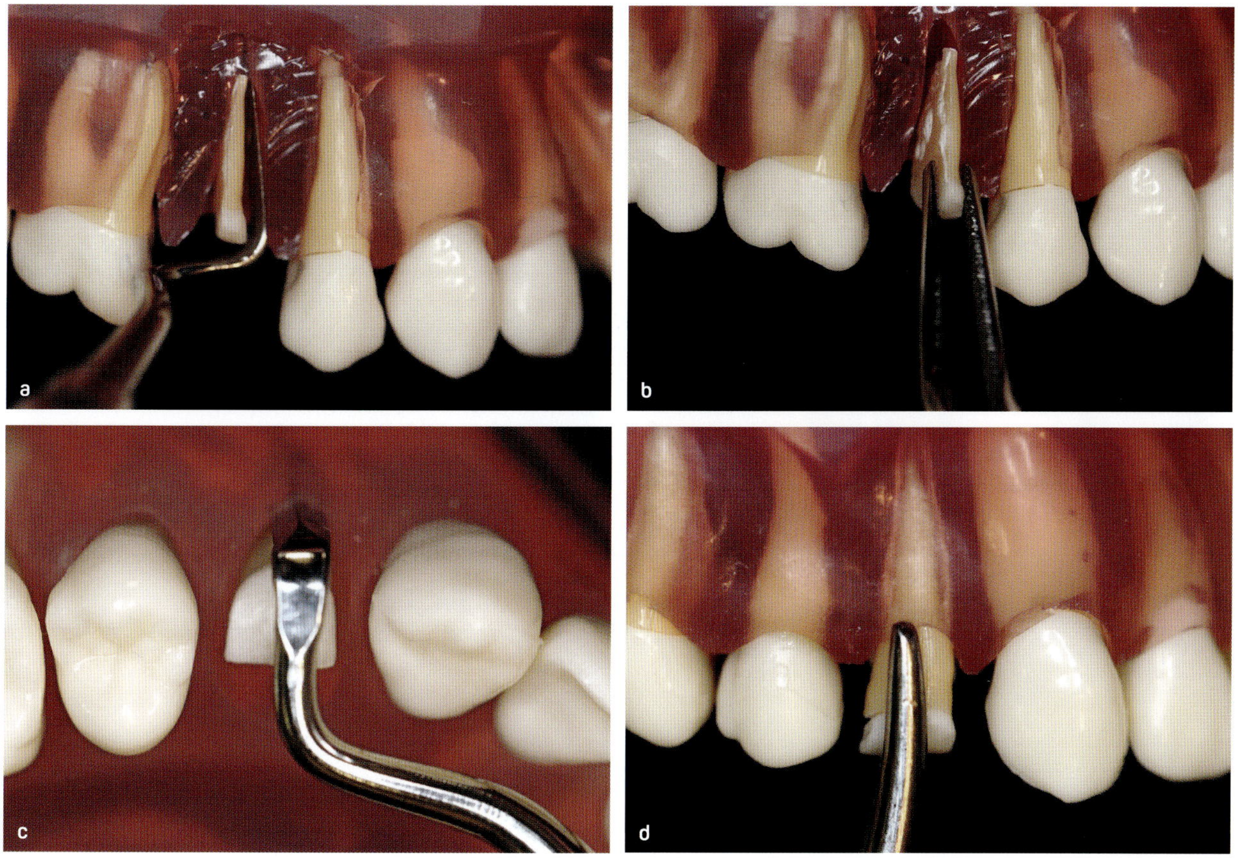

FIG 8-27 *(a)* Using a Hu-Friedy Orban knife K01/2IU to pressure the remaining maxillary right second premolar root section into the space created when the initial half of the root was removed (RSCET). *(b)* Once this remaining root half has been mobilized into the root space, it can be removed with a hemostat or tweezers. *(c)* Hu-Friedy Orban knife K01/2IU used in the buccal sulcus of the maxillary right first premolar to mobilize the remaining buccal root into the space created by removal of the palatal root. Care must be taken because the buccal bone is thin. *(d)* Tweezers are used to remove the buccal root.

Once root segments are mobilized, individual pieces can be removed with a hemostat or tweezers. Lock the hemostat or tweezers onto a mobile root segment as far apically as possible and use a gentle back-and-forth motion with constant pulling pressure to remove the root segment from the socket (Figs 8-25 and 8-26). This technique is helpful in many instances where a tooth fragment has been mobilized and needs to be removed.

After one root section is removed, pressure the remaining root section into the space created by removal of the first (RSCET), and then remove this second root section (Fig 8-27).

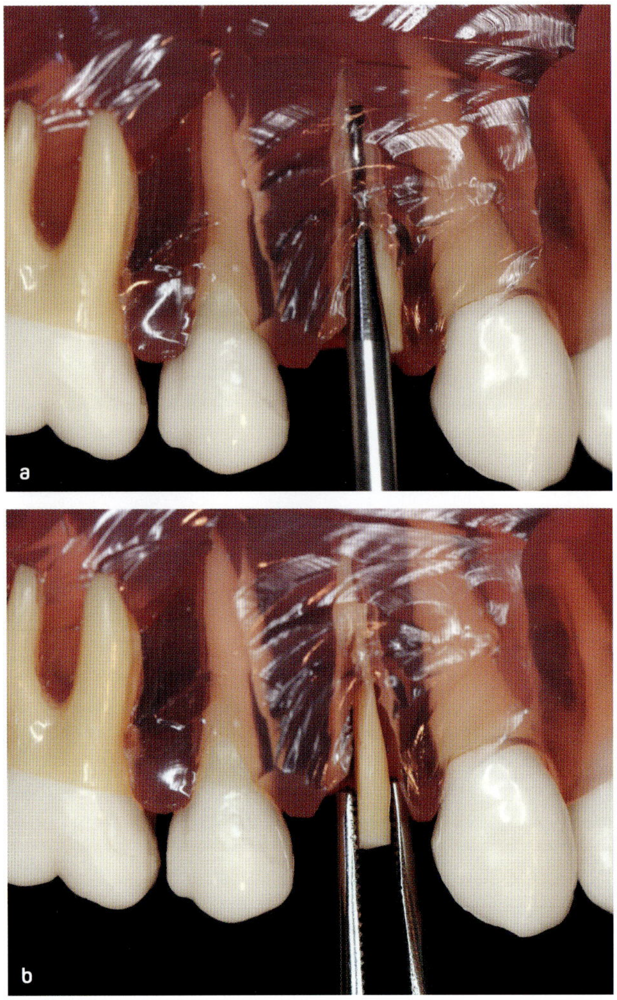

FIG 8-28 *(a)* Buccal root of the maxillary right first premolar being sectioned vertically through the apex with a straight handpiece bur #4 in a buccopalatal direction. *(b)* Mesial half of the buccal root being removed with tweezers.

Section Roots Again; Pressure into Space Created

If the buccal and palatal roots of the maxillary first premolars cannot be removed, you may find that reentering the cut area and sectioning deeper between the roots may be helpful. If this does not work, they must be sectioned again but in a buccopalatal direction (Fig 8-28). It is very important to section all the way through the apex, since luxating two halves of incompletely sectioned roots may result in a fracture coronal to the apex, leaving the root tip connected to one of the sectioned root pieces. If the surgical-length crosscut fissure bur does not reach the apex, use a straight handpiece bur #4 or #6 to cut completely through the apex. This requires opening up the cut wider at the coronal aspect to allow room for the shank of the straight handpiece bur. When the root is completely sectioned through the apex, you will feel the handpiece drop into the softer bone. Cut toward the buccal and palatal slightly to make sure the cut is through the root structure. Then, pressure the root sections into the space created (RSCET) and remove them.

Similarly, if the root halves of the maxillary second premolars cannot be mobilized and removed, consider vertically sectioning one and possibly both root halves so they are in quarters, being careful to avoid the mesial and distal socket walls. This is more applicable to larger roots, but smaller roots may require this step, at which time you are actually drilling out most of the root. Again, it is necessary to drill through the apex; feeling the bur drop into softer bone is an indication that you are past the apex. Then, pressure those root quarters into the space created (RSCET) and remove them.

Once root removal is complete, proceed to socket debridement (see chapter 11).

Complications

If the root is not sectioned entirely through the apex or if the apex fractures, atraumatic removal is difficult. The following steps will help reduce the severity of such complications.

As mentioned earlier, if the root is not sectioned entirely through the apex, pressuring the root into the space may result in a horizontal fracture at the depth of the cut (see Fig 8-19a). If horizontal fracture occurs, remove the loose root fragment (Fig 8-29). The choice is then to attempt to pressure the remaining root, with the apex attached, into the space created by removing the root fragment or to section through the apex.

If the remaining root is pressured into the space created by removing the root fragment (RSCET; Fig 8-30), the risk is another horizontal root fracture, leaving the entire apex. This approach is more successful in softer maxillary bone. Attempting this in the denser mandibular bone will result in fractures more frequently. The other option is to section through the apex (Fig 8-31).

A fractured apex is a complication we will all experience. Sectioning entirely through the apex is necessary to help prevent these complications.

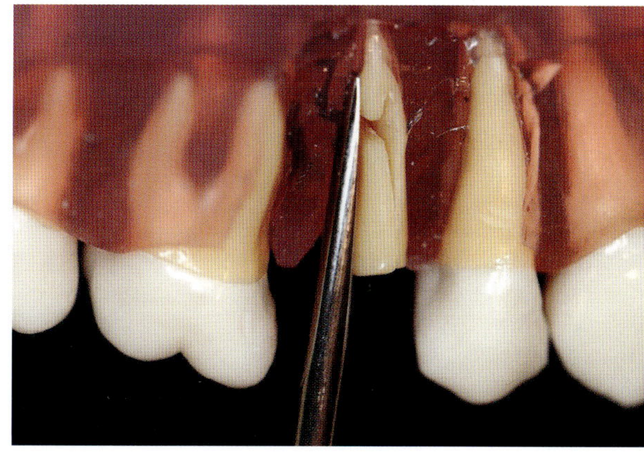

FIG 8-29 If horizontal fracture occurs, the first step is to remove the loose root fragment.

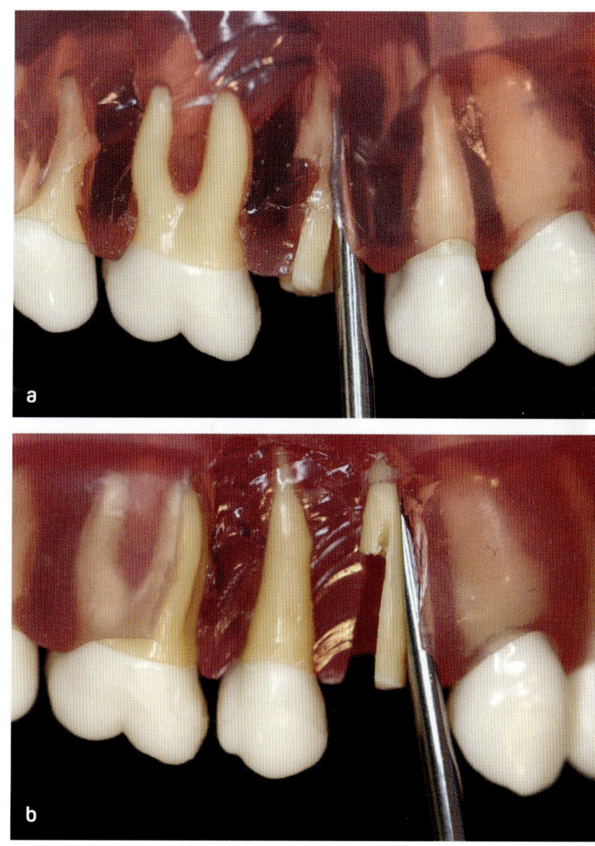

FIG 8-30 *(a)* The thin Directa Luxator L2S elevator is used to pressure the remaining root of the maxillary right second premolar, with apex attached, into the space created by removing the root fragment (RSCET). *(b)* The same thin elevator pressuring the remaining buccal root of the maxillary right first premolar, with apex attached as a result of incomplete buccopalatal sectioning, into the space created by removing the root fragment.

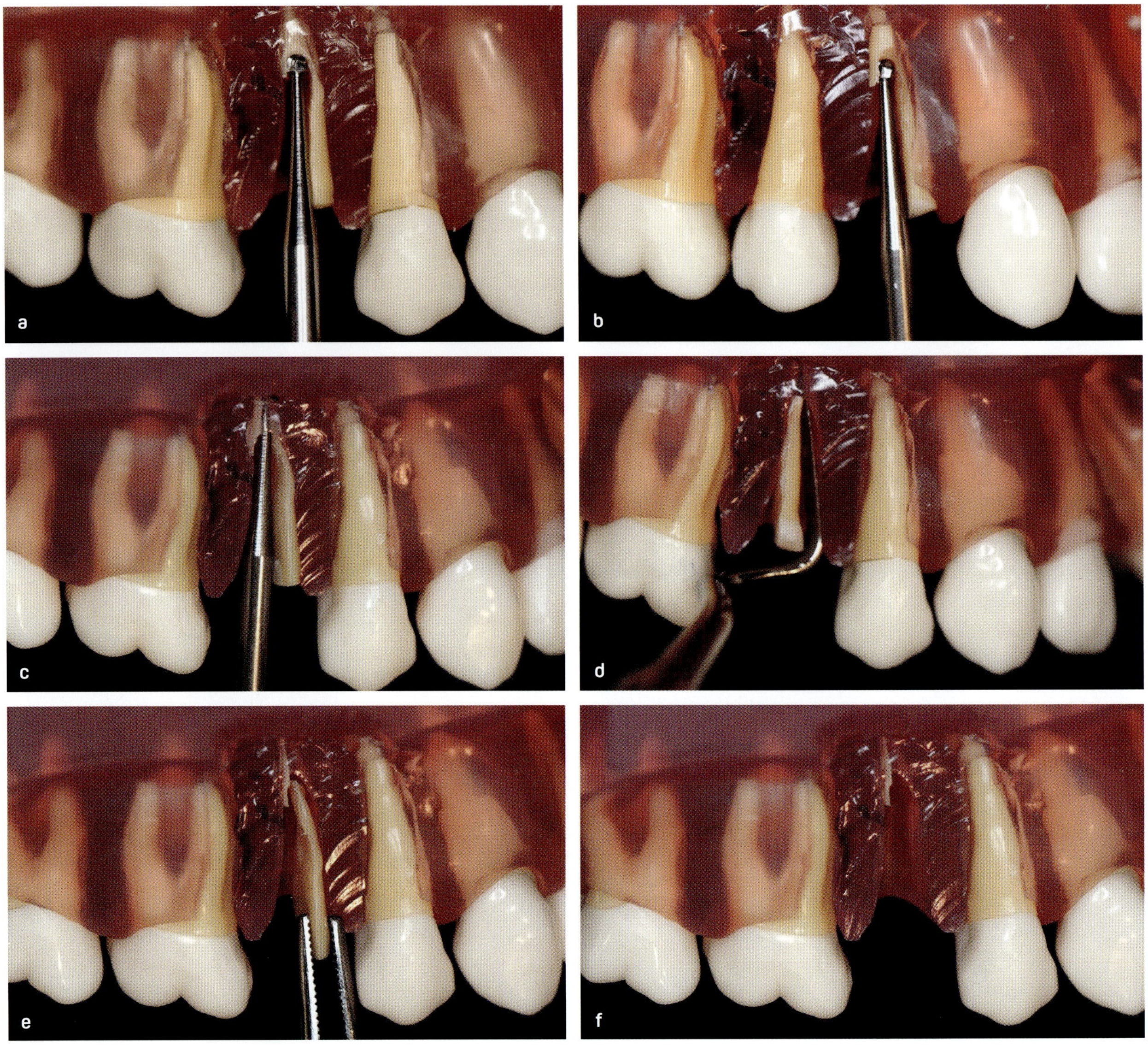

FIG 8-31 *(a)* If horizontal fracture occurs, remove the loose root fragment and use a straight handpiece bur #4 or #6 to completely section the root through the apex (shown on the maxillary right second premolar). *(b)* Same situation shown on the buccal root of the maxillary right first premolar. *(c)* Straight handpiece bur sectioning through the apex of the maxillary right second premolar. *(d)* Once you are through the apex, use the Hu-Friedy Orban knife KO1/2IU to pressure the root half into the space created by removal of the root fragment. *(e)* Remove the long root fragment. *(f)* Half apex remaining. This can be mobilized using a thin elevator and then removed with tweezers or by flushing with sterile saline.

9

Atraumatic Extraction of the Maxillary Molars: Divide and Conquer

The following atraumatic extraction techniques apply to maxillary molars with minimal to no mobility and good bone support. Obviously, teeth with Class II or III mobility can usually be removed atraumatically if there is adequate crown structure to grasp with a forceps. Also, it may not be necessary to use all of the following techniques to atraumatically remove a tooth. Some of the steps may be deemed nonproductive or not applicable to the clinical situation and therefore can be skipped at the discretion of the operating dentist.

Verify Profound Anesthesia

Probe the sulcus with a periodontal probe and stimulate the adjacent gingiva, especially on the palatal, to confirm you have profound anesthesia (Fig 9-1). If anesthesia is inadequate, administer either another nerve block or infiltration into the sulcus and adjacent gingiva circumferentially (Fig 9-2). For quickest onset, use 4% articaine with 1:100,000 epinephrine. For hemostasis, 2% lidocaine 1:100,000 epinephrine is helpful.

A bite block can be used to stabilize the mandible; this also helps patients hold their mouth open during the procedure, reducing muscle fatigue.

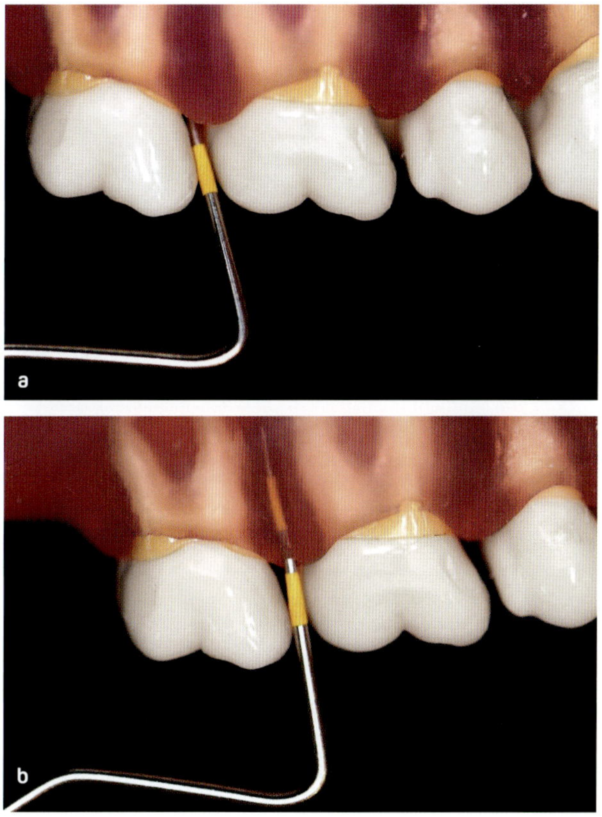

FIG 9-1 Verifying adequate anesthesia. *(a)* Probing the mesiobuccal sulcus of the maxillary right second molar. *(b)* Probing the gingiva between the maxillary right first and second molars.

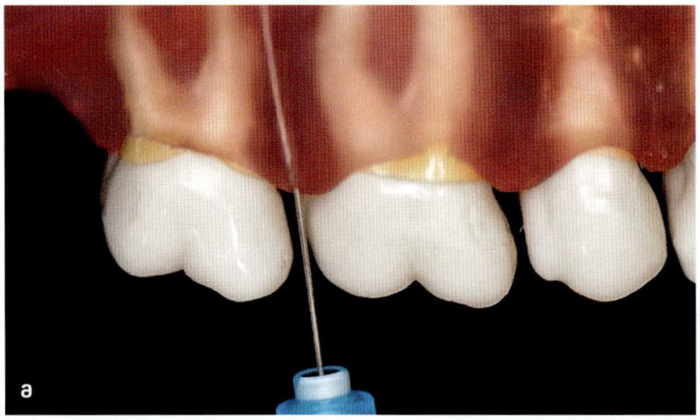
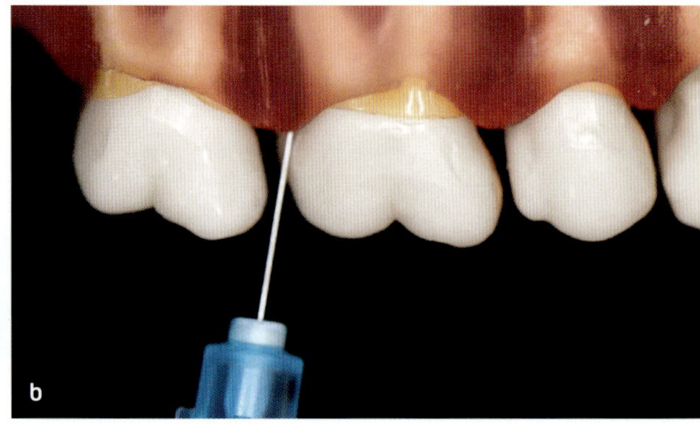

FIG 9-2 Supplementing anesthesia in adjacent gingiva and sulcus. *(a)* Infiltration directly into the papilla between the maxillary right first and second molars. *(b)* Infiltration into the distobuccal sulcus of the maxillary right first molar.

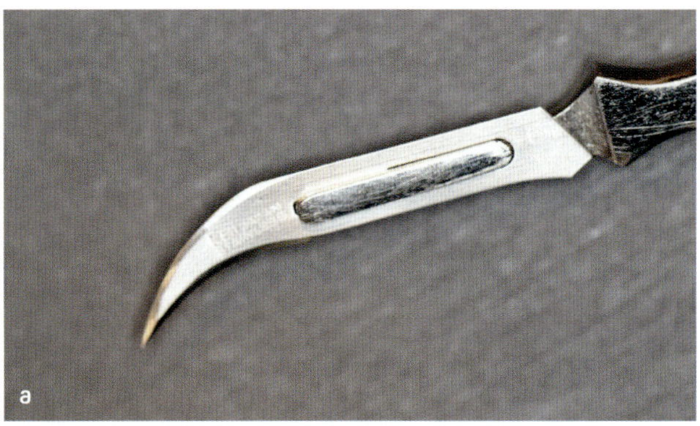
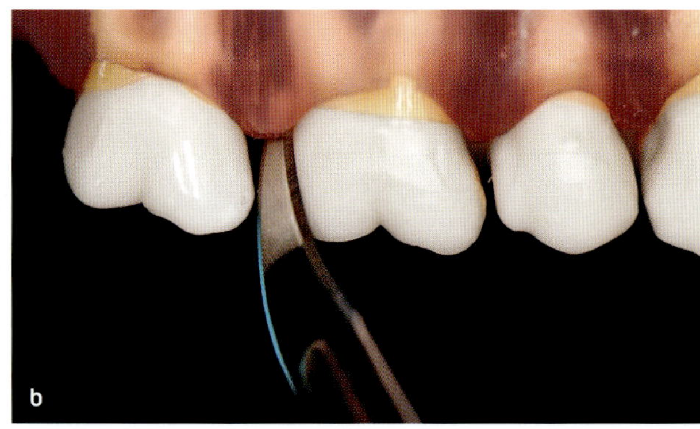

FIG 9-3 *(a)* A 12D scalpel blade. *(b)* The scalpel blade inserted into the distobuccal sulcus of the maxillary right first molar to release the periodontal ligament fibers using a back-and-forth rocking motion with vertical pressure.

Release Periodontal Ligament Fibers Without Flap Reflection

Note that some practitioners remove the crown as the first step. They feel that getting the crown out of the way and just dealing with the root(s) is the most efficient and atraumatic method to remove a tooth. For the purposes of this chapter, we will assume the crown will be left in place for these initial procedures.

Using a 12D scalpel blade, enter the sulcus on the mesial, distal, and palatal, but not the buccal due to the thin buccal bone being vulnerable to resorption and fracture. Apply vertical pressure with a back-and-forth rocking motion (Fig 9-3).

Optional procedure

Use a periotome to excise the periodontal ligament as deeply as possible two times in the mesial, distal, and palatal sulci (Fig 9-4). Avoid the buccal, where the bone is thin. Use a back-and-forth motion with vertical pressure. However, it may be difficult to get into the periodontal ligament space due to lack of space or ankylosis. If that is the case, proceed to the recommended procedure below.

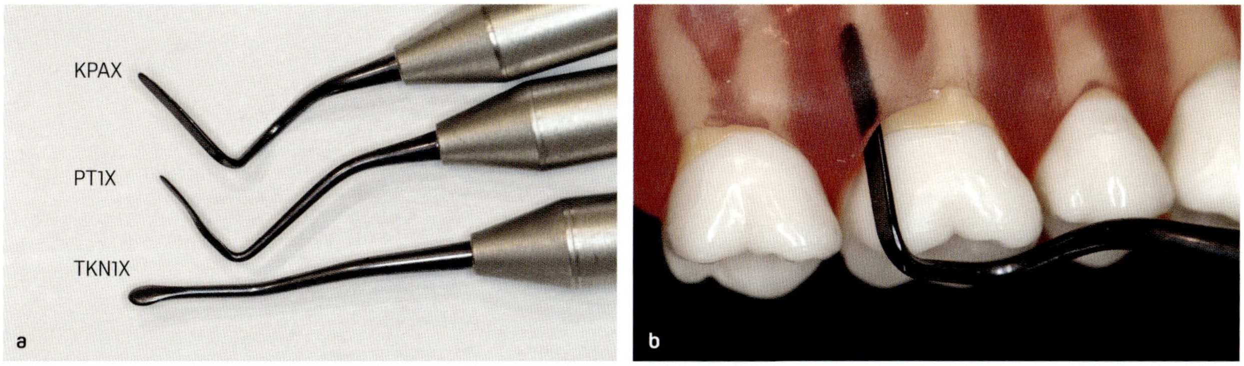

FIG 9-4 *(a)* Hu-Friedy periotomes. *(b)* Periotome inserted into the distobuccal sulcus of the maxillary right first molar to excise periodontal ligament fibers. Use vertical pressure and a back-and-forth rocking motion. Avoid the thin buccal bone.

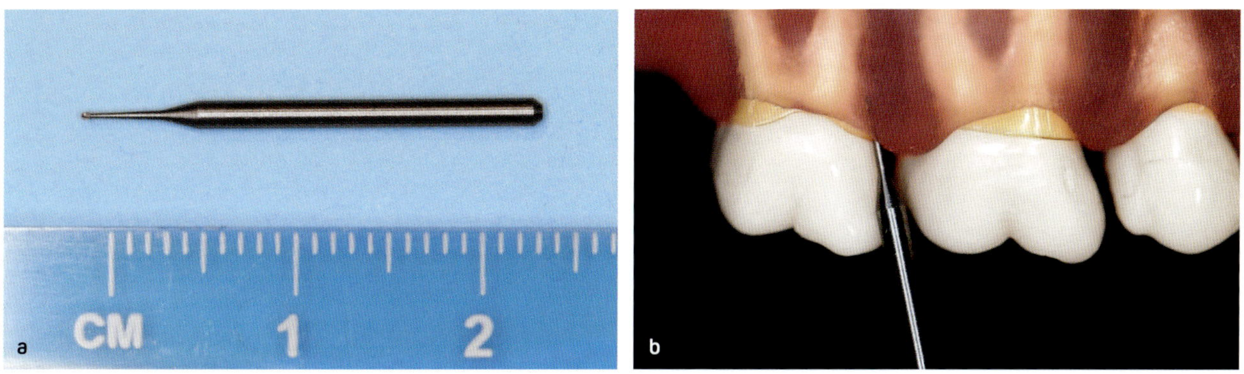

FIG 9-5 *(a)* Surgical-length high-speed ¼ round bur used to separate the root from the bone in the sulcus. *(b)* The bur is inserted in the mesiobuccal sulcus of the maxillary right second molar with an up-and-down pumping motion and light pressure against the root, not the bone.

Recommended procedure

Use a surgical-length high-speed ¼ round bur to further sever the periodontal ligament fibers (Fig 9-5a). Use an up-and-down pumping motion in the periodontal ligament space at the mesial, distal, and palatal, but avoid the buccal since the thin buccal bone is vulnerable to resorption and fracture (Fig 9-5b). Extend as far apically as possible, gently pressuring in the direction of the tooth root rather than the bone of the socket wall. This opening of the periodontal ligament space releases the tooth from the adjacent bone, making it easier to remove, and creates space for a thin elevator to enter and pressure the root.

A periotome, scalpel, or ¼ round high-speed bur may be used in any order.

Attempt Tooth Movement Coronally Without Flap Reflection

Introduce a thin elevator (Fig 9-6) at the mesiobuccal and distobuccal and, using a twisting motion, attempt to move the tooth coronally (Fig 9-7).

If there is adequate crown structure present for luxation of any kind, the following will be helpful.

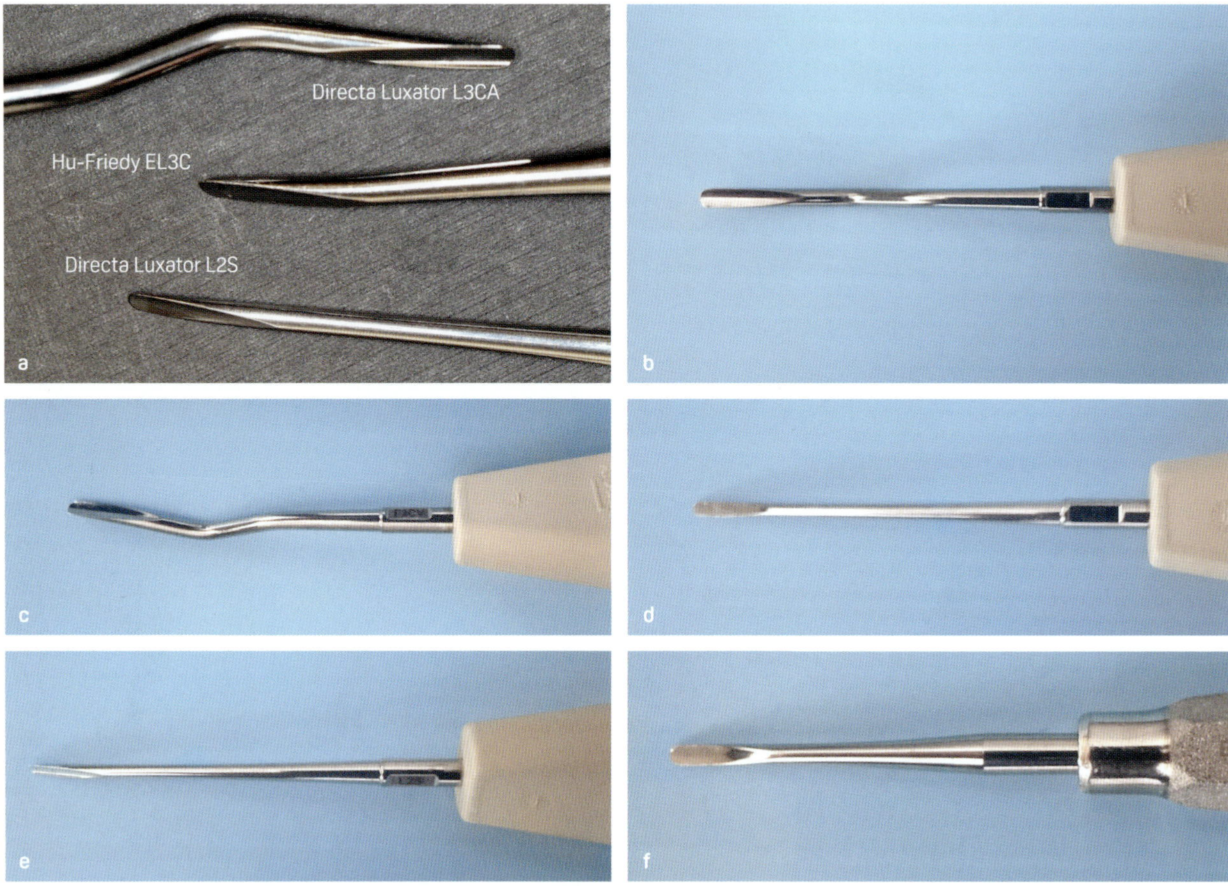

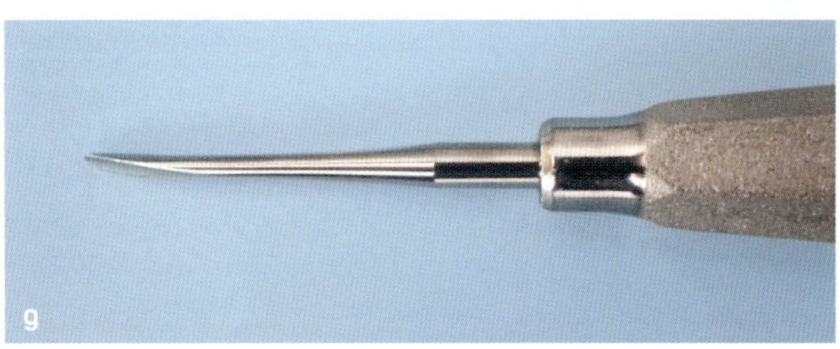

FIG 9-6 *(a)* Examples of thin elevators. *(b)* Directa Luxator L3CA top view. *(c)* Directa Luxator L3CA side view. *(d)* Directa Luxator L2S top view. *(e)* Directa Luxator L2S side view. *(f)* Hu-Friedy EL3C top view. *(g)* Hu-Friedy EL3C side view.

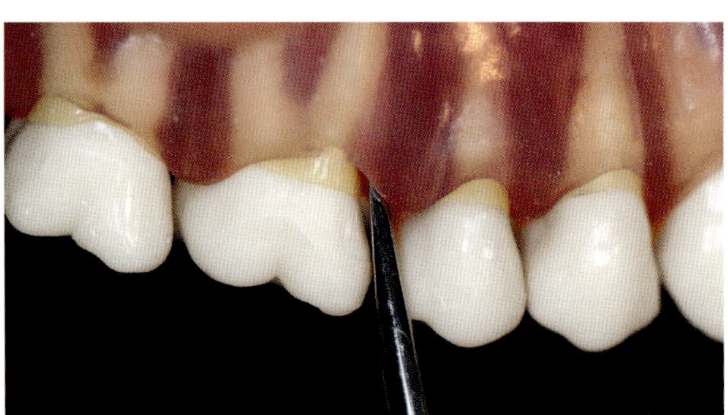

FIG 9-7 Hu-Friedy EL3C elevator inserted in the mesial sulcus of the maxillary right first molar.

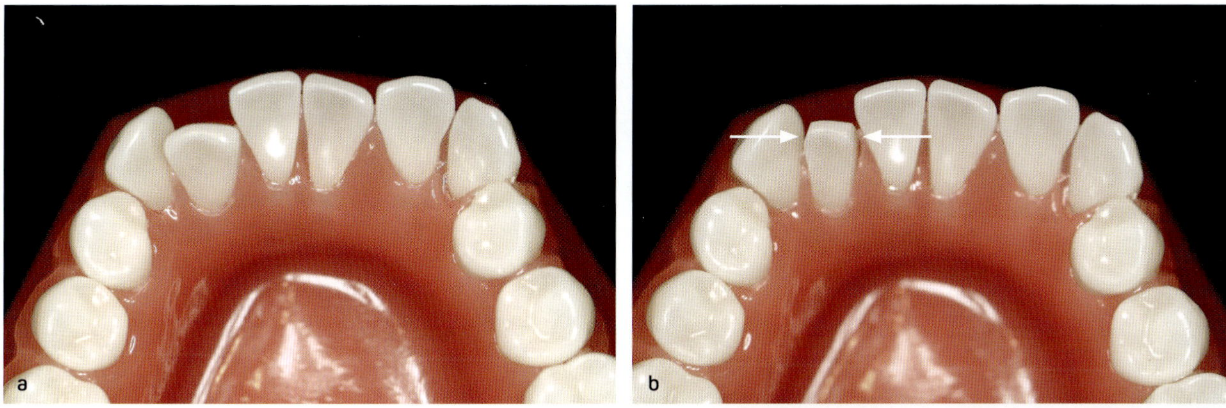

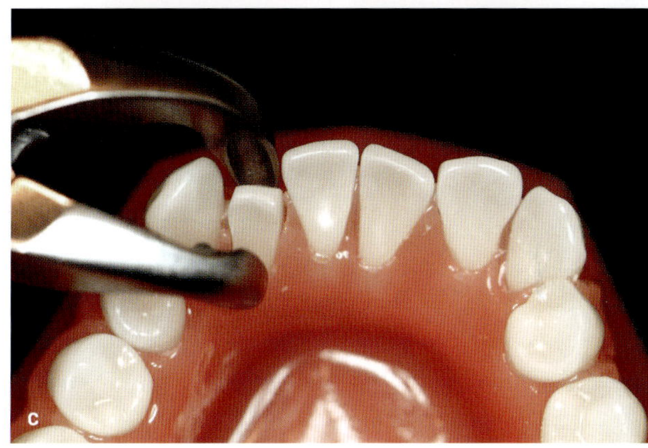

FIG 9-8 *(a)* Mandibular left lateral incisor overlapped with the adjacent canine and central incisor. Rotating the lateral incisor with a forceps will apply pressure to (and may cause increased mobility of) these adjacent teeth. *(b)* The mesial and distal contacts of the lateral incisor have been reduced. *(c)* Now rotation of the lateral incisor with a forceps will be less harmful to adjacent teeth.

Reduce Interproximal Contacts

We are attempting to remove a tooth as atraumatically as possible, and this pertains not only to the tooth being extracted but also to the adjacent teeth, their restorations, and the rest of the mouth as well. If we were to luxate a tooth with tight or overlapping contacts, we would be pressuring the adjacent contacts and therefore moving the adjacent teeth. (If multiple adjacent teeth are being removed, this concept does not apply; luxation of a tooth with tight or overlapping contacts may actually help loosen adjacent teeth planned for extraction.) Therefore, where teeth are overlapped or crowded, I feel it is important to reduce the interproximal contacts on a single tooth to be removed. Note that if interproximal contacts are present, but luxation does not move or harm adjacent teeth or restorations, then reduction of interproximal contacts is not necessary. If contacts are overlapping on one side only, rotate the tooth in the direction that does not increase contact pressure. Figure 9-8 presents overlapping mandibular incisors as an example.

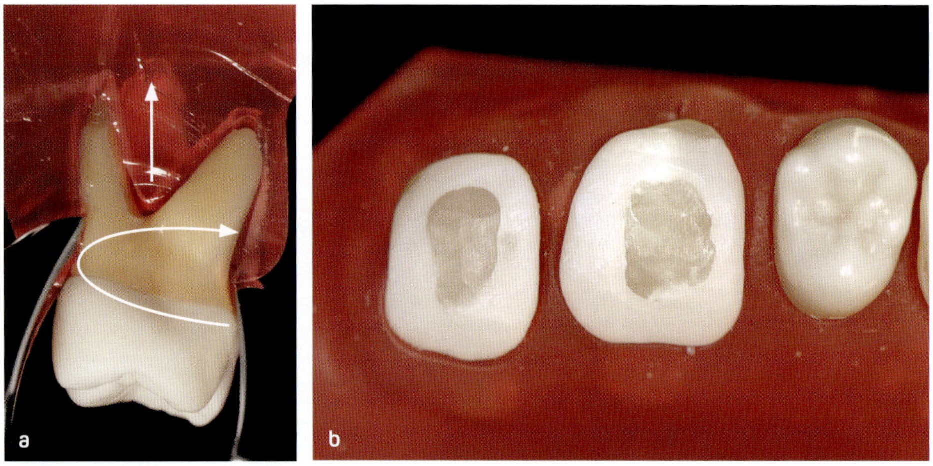

FIG 9-9 *(a)* Forceps applied as far apically as possible without damaging bone or soft tissue. First apply vertical pressure, then rotational movement. *(b)* Crowns removed to show trapezoidal shape of maxillary molars. Excessive rotation may fracture the socket wall or roots.

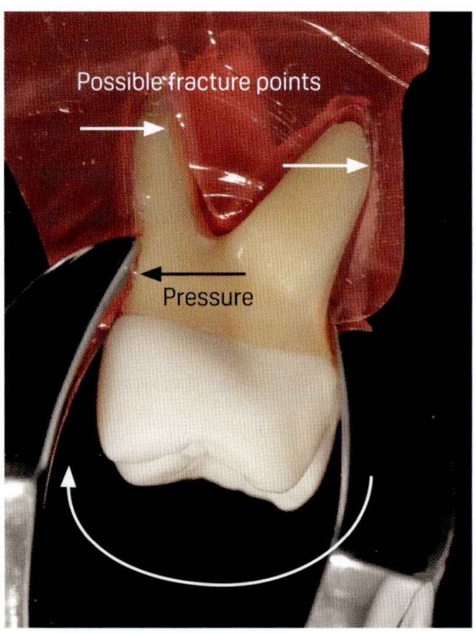

FIG 9-10 Pressure applied coronally toward the buccal of the maxillary right first molar, which also pressures the palatal surfaces of the palatal and buccal roots. This may result in fracture of the apices.

Luxate Gently with Forceps

To gently luxate the tooth, place forceps as far apically as possible without engaging bone. Try to engage the root surface apical to any restoration margins. Gently apply pressure apically and hold for 30 seconds. While continuing to apply apical pressure, gently luxate in a buccal and palatal direction with slight rotation to test the mobility of the tooth (Fig 9-9a). The reason for applying apical pressure while luxating is that it shifts the axis of rotation in an apical direction, reducing the chance for root fracture. Remember, the maxillary molars are trapezoidal in shape (Fig 9-9b). It is recommended to avoid excessive rotation since this will expand the socket and may fracture the socket wall or roots.

If the bone on the buccal or palatal alveolar crest is especially thick, pressure can be placed in that direction. However, it is important to realize that when applying pressure coronally in a lateral direction toward the alveolar crest, the apical portion of the tooth will be forced against the opposite socket wall. This pressure can lead to fracture of one or more root apices, which would have to be retrieved (Fig 9-10). Mandibular bone is denser than maxillary bone; therefore, root fracture is more probable in the mandible, depending on the root anatomy.

If the crown is intact and all three roots are fused, a forceps can be used to remove the tooth. However, if all three roots are not fused, the buccal roots will draw at different angles, and not separating them may damage the surrounding bone or fracture one or more of the roots. Separating them allows them to be removed individually at the angle that causes the least amount of damage to the bone. Therefore, if gentle luxation is not successful in removing the tooth, and the buccal roots are separate from the palatal root with the crown intact, a technique in

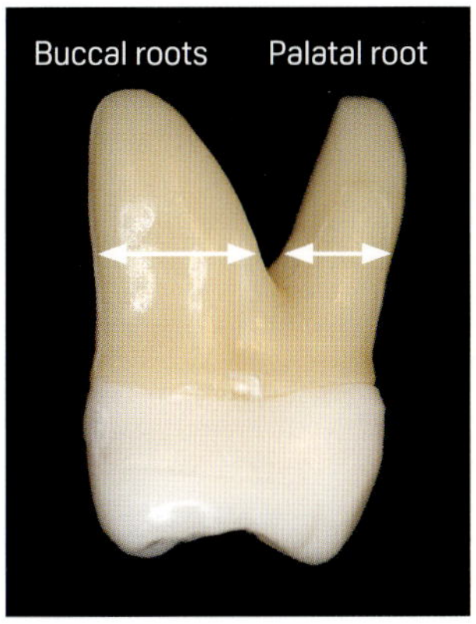

FIG 9-11 Maxillary right first molar viewed from the distal.

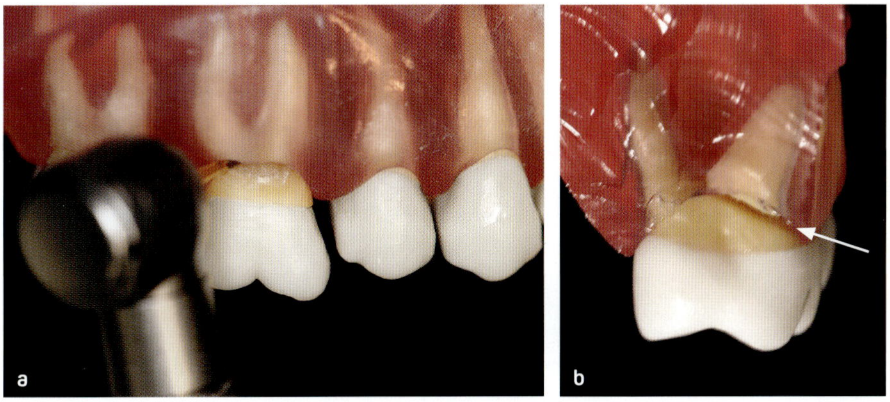

FIG 9-12 *(a)* Using a Great White (SS White) high-speed crosscut fissure bur to horizontally section the buccal roots from the crown, leaving the palatal root attached to the crown. Sectioning must extend approximately two-thirds of the way under the crown in a palatal direction to completely section the buccal roots. *(b)* Distal view of the maxillary right first molar after both buccal roots have been sectioned from the crown. The palatal root is still attached to the crown.

which the crown is sectioned from the buccal roots but left attached to the palatal root (described in the next section) may be useful. In other anatomical situations, it may be best to section the crown from all three roots horizontally about 1 mm coronal to the gingival margin as described under the heading "Section Crown Horizontally at the Cementoenamel Junction" on page 101.

Section Crown from Buccal Roots Only

This technique uses the crown attached to the palatal root as leverage to remove the palatal root. If the roots are sectioned from each other, the palatal root is often the most difficult of the three to remove, so this technique helps alleviate this challenge. Note the larger buccolingual width of the buccal roots versus the palatal root (Fig 9-11).

To completely section the buccal roots from the crown, you will need to section approximately two-thirds of the way under the crown in a palatal direction (Fig 9-12). Once sectioning is complete, use forceps to luxate the crown with a twisting motion, rotating around the axis of the palatal root (Fig 9-13a). As mentioned above, reduction of contacts on the crown to be luxated may be required to prevent moving or damaging the adjacent teeth. This technique usually results in the removal or at least the mobilization of the palatal root attached to the crown, leaving the buccal roots in place (Figs 9-13b to 9-13d).

The remaining buccal roots are then separated if necessary (Fig 9-14a). A thin elevator, periotome, or surgical-length high-speed ¼ round bur is used to mobilize and remove the buccal roots (Figs 9-14b and 9-14c). See "Section Between Non-Fused Roots" on page 103 and the subsequent sections for more details on sectioning, mobilizing, elevating, and removing individual roots (and root fragments if further sectioning is required).

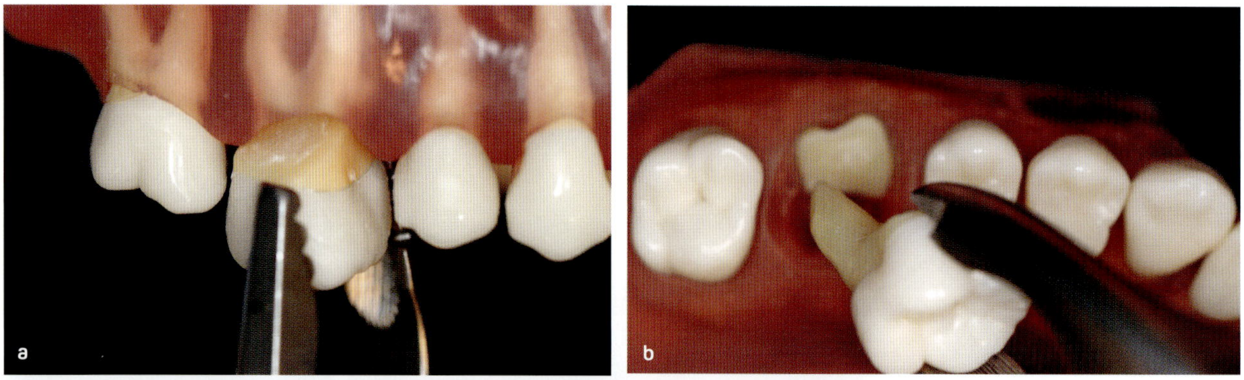

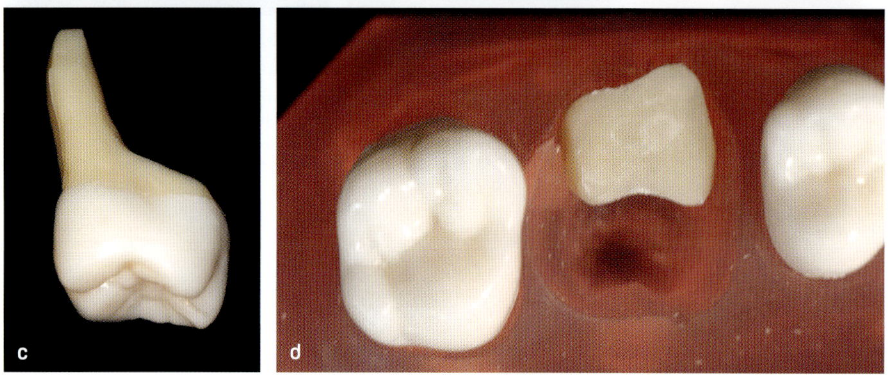

FIG 9-13 *(a)* Using forceps, luxate the crown in a twisting motion, rotating around the axis of the palatal root. *(b and c)* The maxillary right first molar crown is removed with the palatal root attached, leaving the buccal roots in place. *(d)* The remaining buccal roots are attached at their coronal aspect.

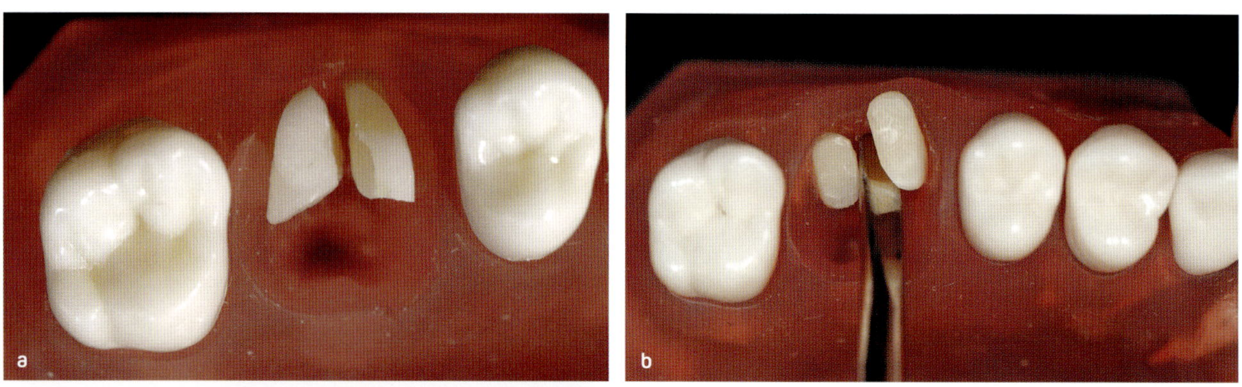

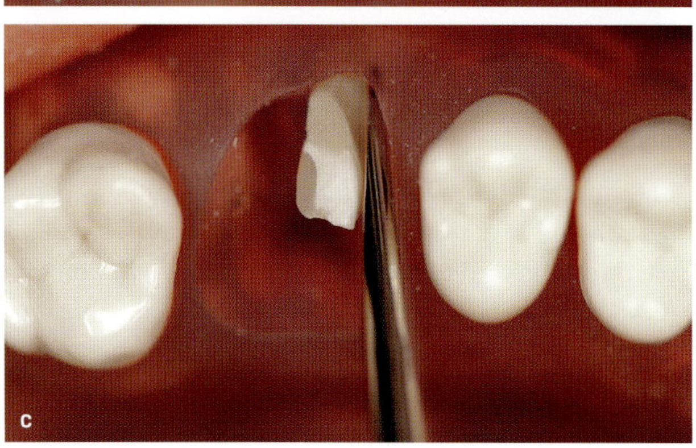

FIG 9-14 *(a)* Buccal roots sectioned into individual roots. *(b)* Hu-Friedy EL3C elevator pressuring between the separated roots and mobilizing them. *(c)* Same elevator used to pressure the mesiobuccal root into the space created by removal of the distobuccal root.

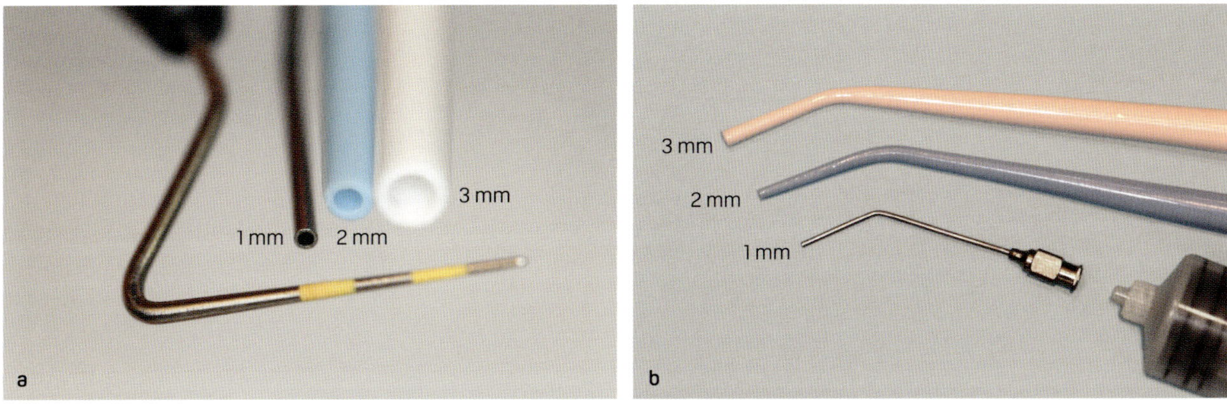

FIG 9-15 *(a and b)* Thin 1-mm irrigation tip and 2- and 3-mm-diameter suction tips used during sectioning of a crown.

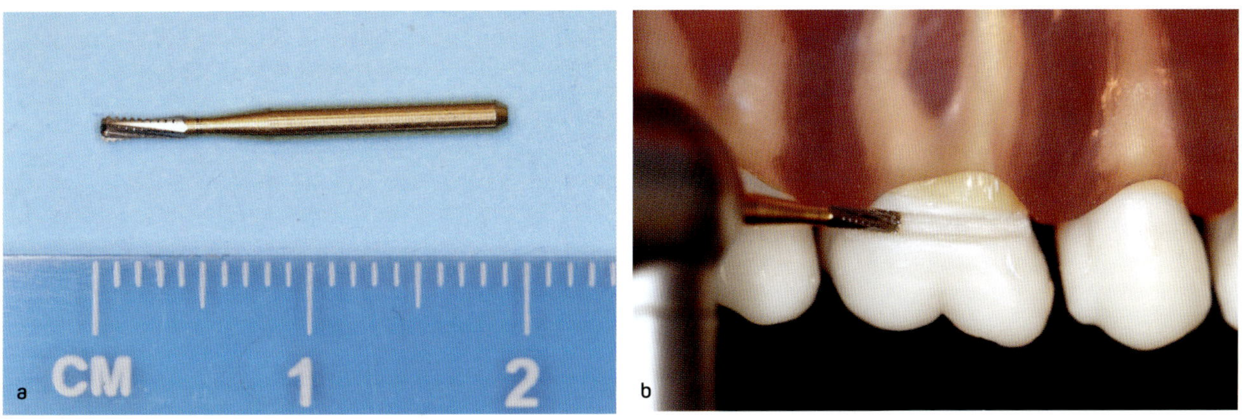

FIG 9-16 *(a)* Great White high-speed crosscut fissure bur used to horizontally section the crown. *(b)* Sectioning the maxillary right first molar crown 1 mm coronal to the free gingival margin.

Section Crown Horizontally at the Cementoenamel Junction

This technique can be used for maxillary molars with fused or non-fused roots. Some practitioners go right to this step for every extraction, feeling that it is the most efficient and atraumatic method.

When sectioning a crown or roots, it is important to use plenty of saline irrigation with a thin irrigation tip to remove tooth debris and to use a thin suction tip to suction within the drill cuts and sockets. This allows you to see and feel in these areas (Fig 9-15). Section the crown 1 mm coronal to the gingival margin using a Great White high-speed crosscut fissure bur (Fig 9-16). It is important to be aware of the gingival margin location to avoid lacerating the gingiva. Leaving the root 1 mm above the gingival margin allows a starting point for a thin elevator, surgical-length ¼ round bur, or periotome to enter the sulcus to pressure the root.

Obviously, it's much easier to section through tooth structure or a composite restoration as compared to a metal restoration. Regardless of the material, section two-thirds of the way through the crown, and then, using an elevator, gently pry off the crown. Using a football-shaped high-speed diamond bur, smooth the

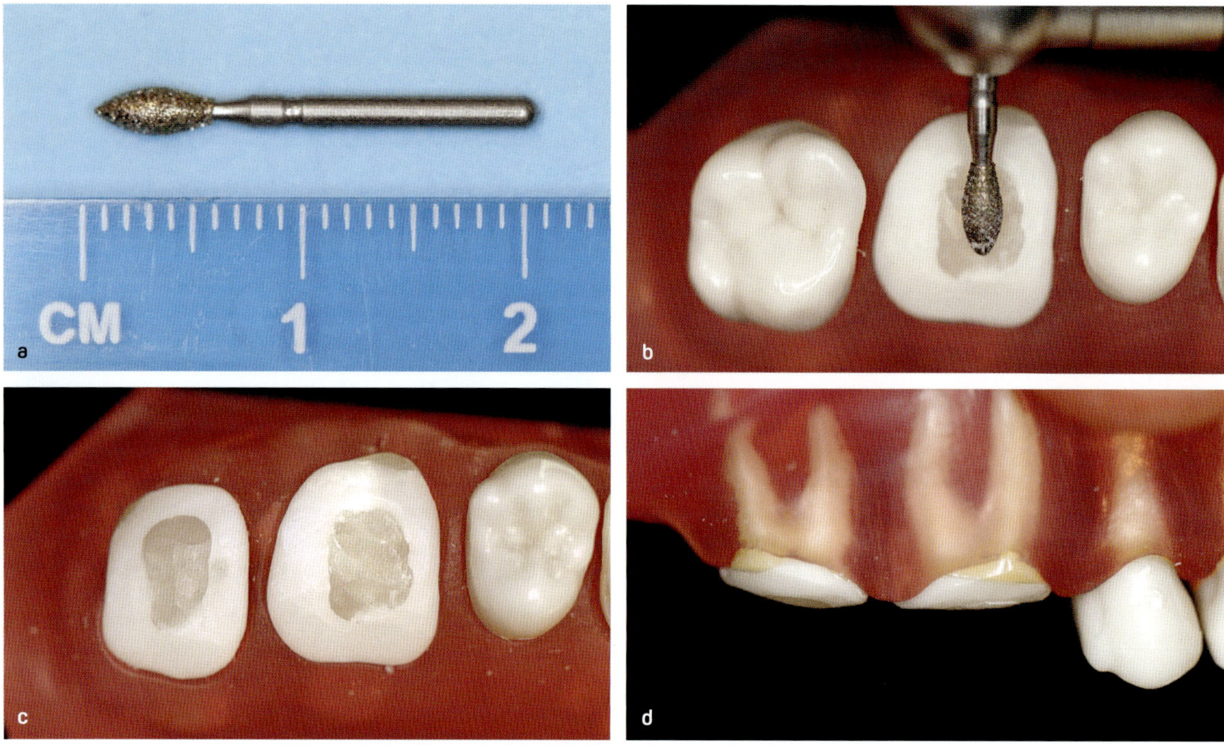

FIG 9-17 *(a)* High-speed football diamond bur used to smooth the remaining root to a level 1 mm above the gingival margin after sectioning off the crown. *(b)* Bur used to smooth the remaining root of the maxillary right first molar. *(c and d)* Occlusal and buccal views of the maxillary right first and second molars sectioned 1 mm above the gingival margin.

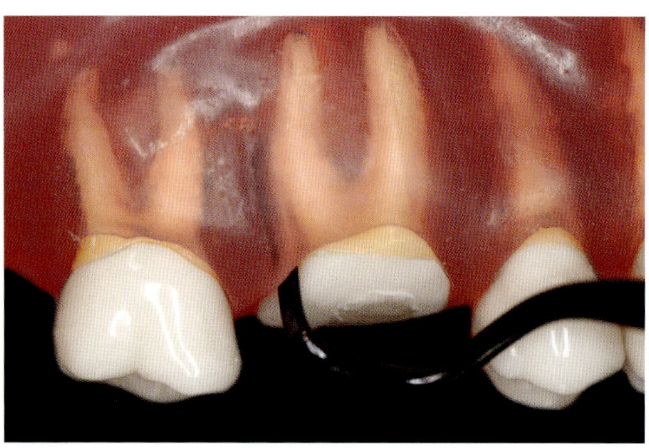

FIG 9-18 Periotome in the distal sulcus of the maxillary right first molar using vertical pressure and a back-and-forth rocking motion. Avoid the buccal, where bone is thin.

remaining tooth structure to a fairly flat surface approximately 1 mm coronal to the gingival margin (Fig 9-17).

Some maxillary second and third molars have fused roots. If the roots are not fused, they can be easier to remove if they are sectioned from each other. Removing the crown allows you to see the remaining root structure, including where the roots divide, and to determine the best location to section vertically. Vertical fractures may be evident also. A dye such as To Dye For (Roydent) may be used to help visualize possible fractures.

Optional procedure

Release the periodontal ligament fibers again using a narrow periotome. Enter the sulcus on the palatal, mesial, and distal, applying vertical pressure and a back-and-forth rocking motion to excise the periodontal ligament fibers further apically (Fig 9-18).

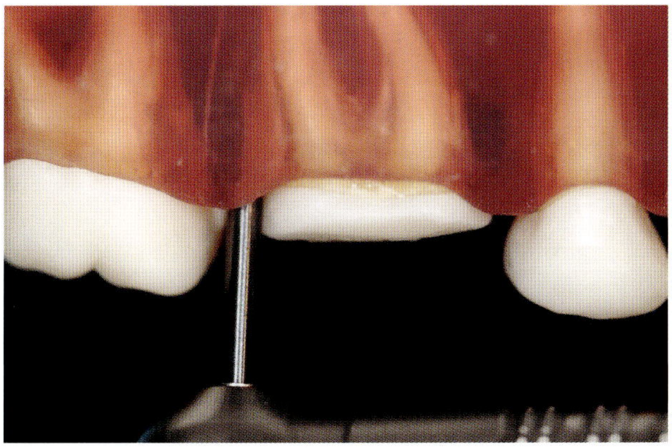

FIG 9-19 Surgical-length ¼ round high-speed bur used with a gentle up-and-down motion in the distobuccal sulcus of the maxillary right first molar, exerting pressure toward the root, not the bone of the socket wall.

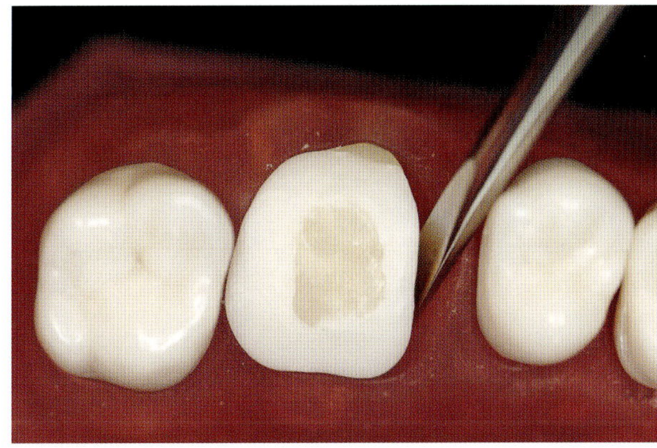

FIG 9-20 A thin elevator is used to gently luxate the tooth with a twisting motion, attempting to mobilize it.

Recommended procedure

Instead of a periotome, you can use a surgical-length ¼ round high-speed bur to further sever the periodontal ligament fibers (Fig 9-19). Attempt to cut more in the direction of the root rather than the bone of the socket wall. Excising periodontal ligament fibers like this detaches the root from the bone, allowing for easier extraction. Avoid the buccal aspect because bone in this area is thin.

Use Thin Elevator to Mobilize Tooth Without Flap Reflection

Introducing a thin elevator (see Fig 9-6a) at the mesiobuccal and distobuccal, use a twisting motion to attempt to move the tooth coronally (Fig 9-20). This is done to begin mobilizing the tooth.

Section Between Non-Fused Roots

The most atraumatic technique for removing a maxillary molar with non-fused roots is to separate the roots from each other, since each root draws in a different direction. If an attempt is made to remove the tooth in one piece, one or more of the roots may fracture and bone may be damaged in the process.

Evaluate the radiographic appearance of the roots to determine the depth of cut required to separate them. Be aware that the maxillary sinus is usually close to the maxillary molar roots. The sinus may be situated in the roof of the furcation between the roots. Therefore, when sectioning the roots, be aware that the bur may enter the maxillary sinus. Use a surgical-length high-speed crosscut bur (Fig 9-21a) and section in a Y pattern, being careful to cut only tooth structure and minimize bone damage as much as possible. Section between both buccal roots and then separate the distobuccal and mesiobuccal roots from the palatal root (Figs 9-21b and 9-21c).

This technique is termed the *root space creation extraction technique* (*RSCET*). The concept involves using a bur to remove tooth structure and creating a space into which the divided roots can be pressured, away from the sulcus and socket wall. In this way, tooth roots can be removed without removing supporting bone. It is important that you have thin sterile saline irrigation and suction tips that reach the apices of the roots you are sectioning, allowing you to irrigate and suction the drill cuts, removing tooth debris for visualization.

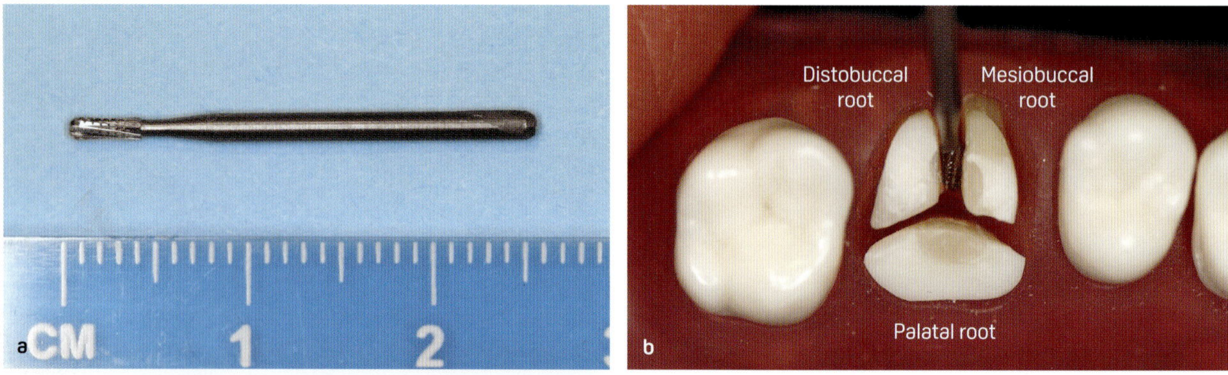

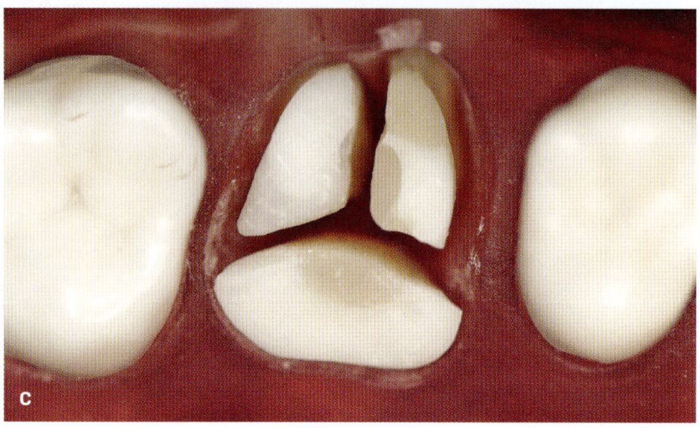

FIG 9-21 *(a)* Surgical-length high-speed crosscut fissure bur. *(b and c)* The bur is used to section between the maxillary right first molar roots in a Y pattern, separating the distobuccal, mesiobuccal, and palatal roots.

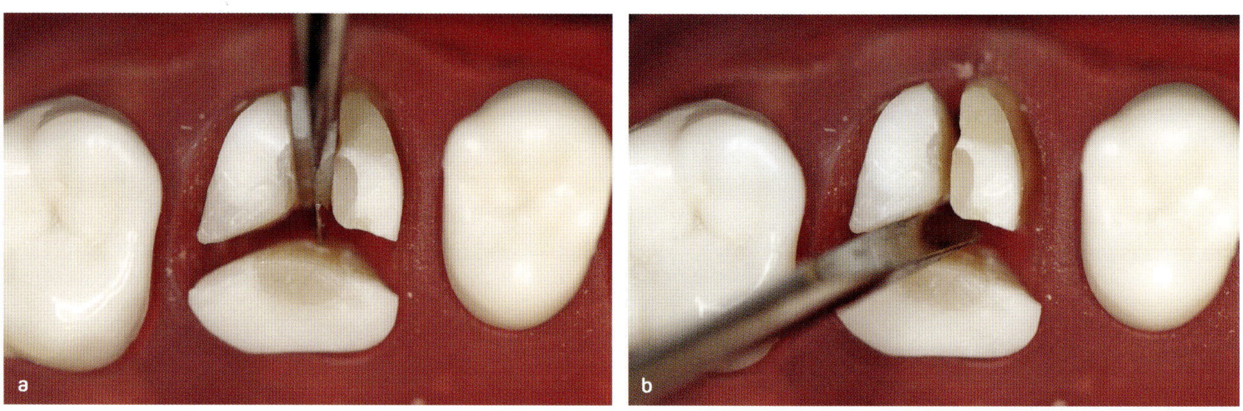

FIG 9-22 *(a and b)* Using the thin Hu-Friedy EL3C elevator to gently pressure and mobilize the roots.

Elevate Gently Between Roots

Introduce an elevator between the sectioned roots and, using a gentle twisting motion, pressure the roots laterally (Fig 9-22). Be aware that you are also pressuring the bone laterally, so if it looks like there is a weak area, avoid pressuring that area.

If pressuring between the roots does not mobilize them, use a periotome or surgical-length high-speed ¼ round bur to further excise the periodontal ligament fibers in the sulcus from the surfaces of the roots. Cut more in the direction of the root, not the bone of the socket wall.

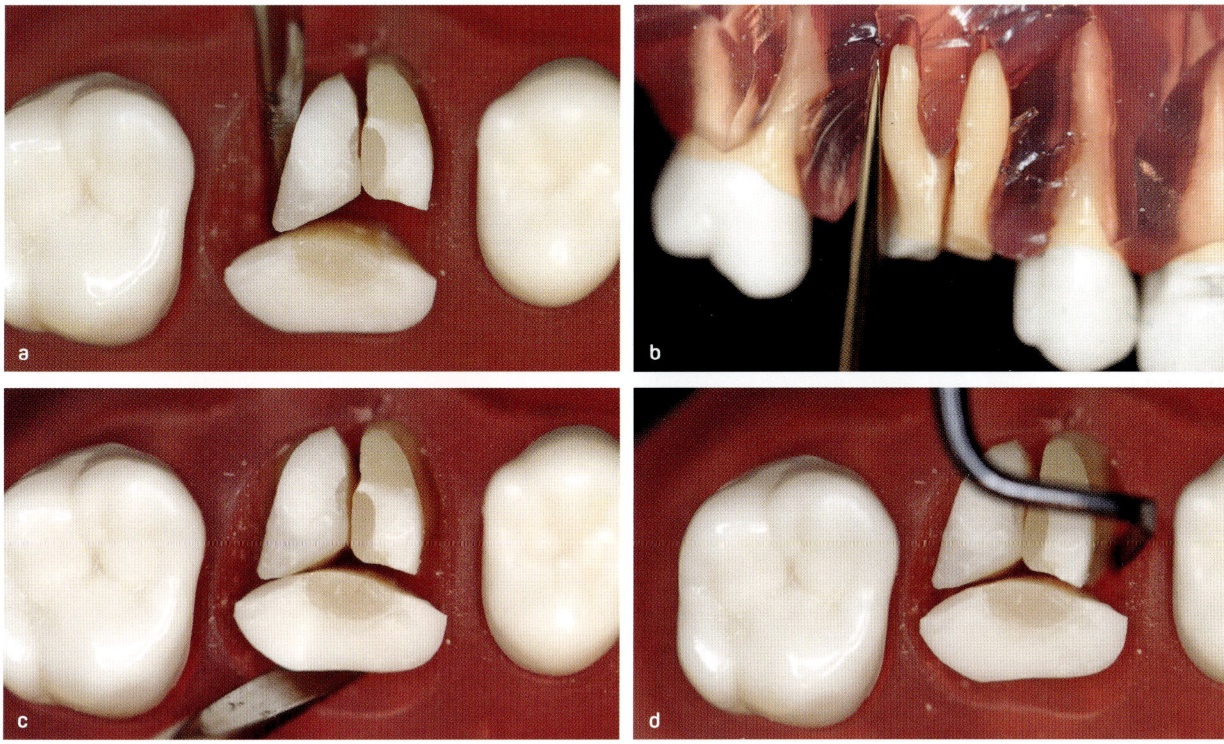

FIG 9-23 *(a and b)* Pressuring the distobuccal root mesially with a thin elevator. *(c)* Pressuring the palatal root buccally. *(d)* Pressuring the mesiobuccal root distally.

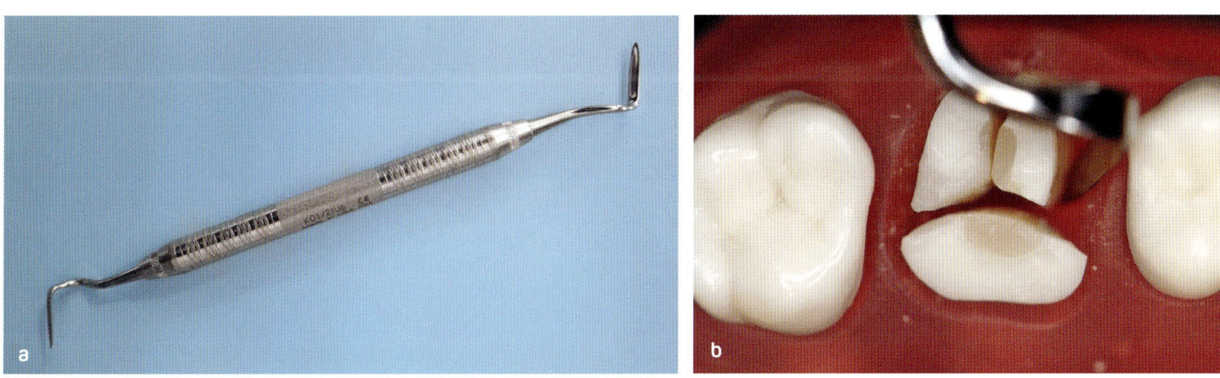

FIG 9-24 *(a)* Hu-Friedy Orban knife KO1/2IU. *(b)* The knife is used to pressure the mesiobuccal root distally.

Enter Sulcus Laterally and Pressure Roots into Sectioned Space

Insert a thin elevator or Hu-Friedy Orban knife KO1/2IU into the sulcus and pressure the roots into the space created by sectioning the roots. This involves pressuring the mesiobuccal root distally or distopalatally, the distobuccal root mesially or mesiopalatally, and the palatal root buccally, mesiobuccally, or distobuccally (Figs 9-23 and 9-24). It is important to insert the instrument as far apically as possible and pressure the root laterally, not tilting the instrument, which could cause the root tips to fracture.

Once the roots are mobilized, individual roots can be removed with a hemostat or tweezers. Lock the hemostat or tweezers onto a mobile root as far apically as possible and use a gentle back-and-forth motion with constant pulling pressure to remove the root from the

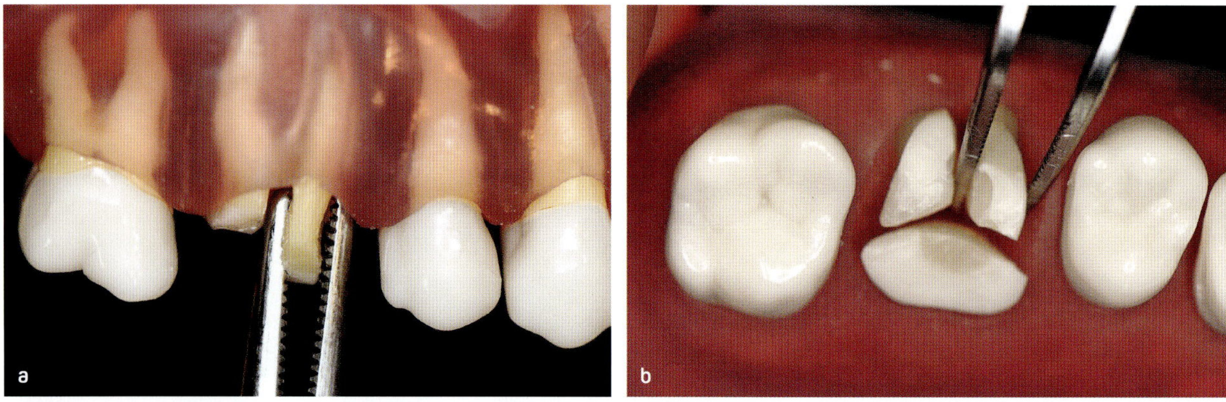

FIG 9-25 *(a)* Hemostat locked onto the mesiobuccal root of the maxillary right first molar, using a back-and-forth motion and constant pulling pressure to remove it from the socket. *(b)* Removing the mobilized mesiobuccal root with tweezers.

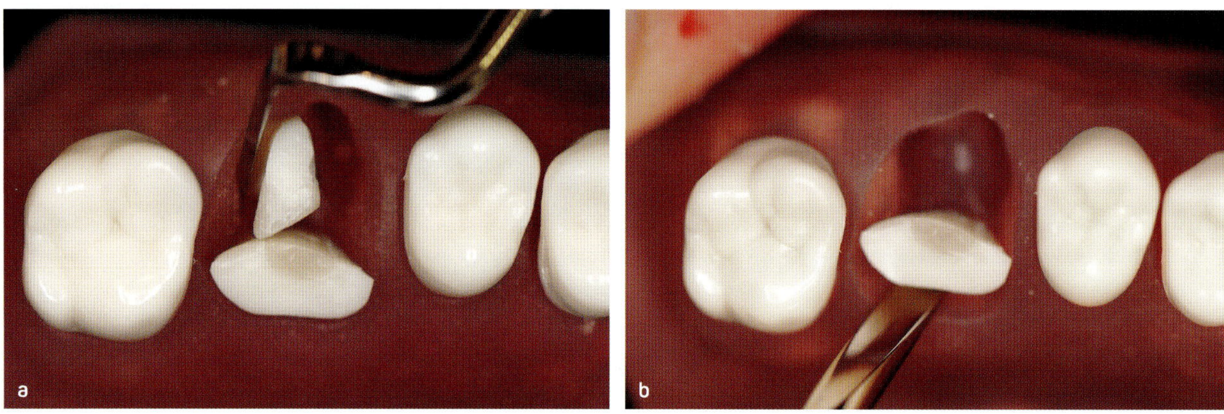

FIG 9-26 *(a)* Distobuccal root being pressured into the space created by removal of the mesiobuccal root. *(b)* Remaining palatal root being pressured into the space created by removal of both buccal roots.

socket (Fig 9-25). This technique is helpful in many instances where a tooth fragment has been mobilized and needs to be removed.

If this is not successful, reenter the sulcus with a periotome, surgical-length high-speed ¼ round bur, or thin elevator. Once again, excise the periodontal ligament fibers and try to pressure the roots into the space created between them.

Once one of the three maxillary molar roots is removed, pressure one of the other roots into the adjacent space created by removal of the first root (Fig 9-26a). When two of the three roots have been removed, pressure the last root into the space that exhibits the least resistance (Fig 9-26b).

Another option is to use the Easy X-Trac System (A. Titan) or Benex Root Extraction System (Meisinger) (see chapter 12). For maxillary molars, the palatal root is the only root large enough to be removed with these systems, both of which involve drilling a hole down the middle of the root canal space and inserting a threaded rod. This rod is pulled coronally with a wedging device, removing the root in one piece. Since the root is tapered, there is minimal trauma when it is removed in a vertical direction with the Easy X-Trac or Benex.

Section Roots Themselves; Elevate Gently Between Root Fragments

If elevation and removal of the individual roots is not successful, then sectioning of the roots themselves is indicated. As before, use thin irrigation and suction tips that reach the apex of the roots you are sectioning to irrigate and suction drill cuts.

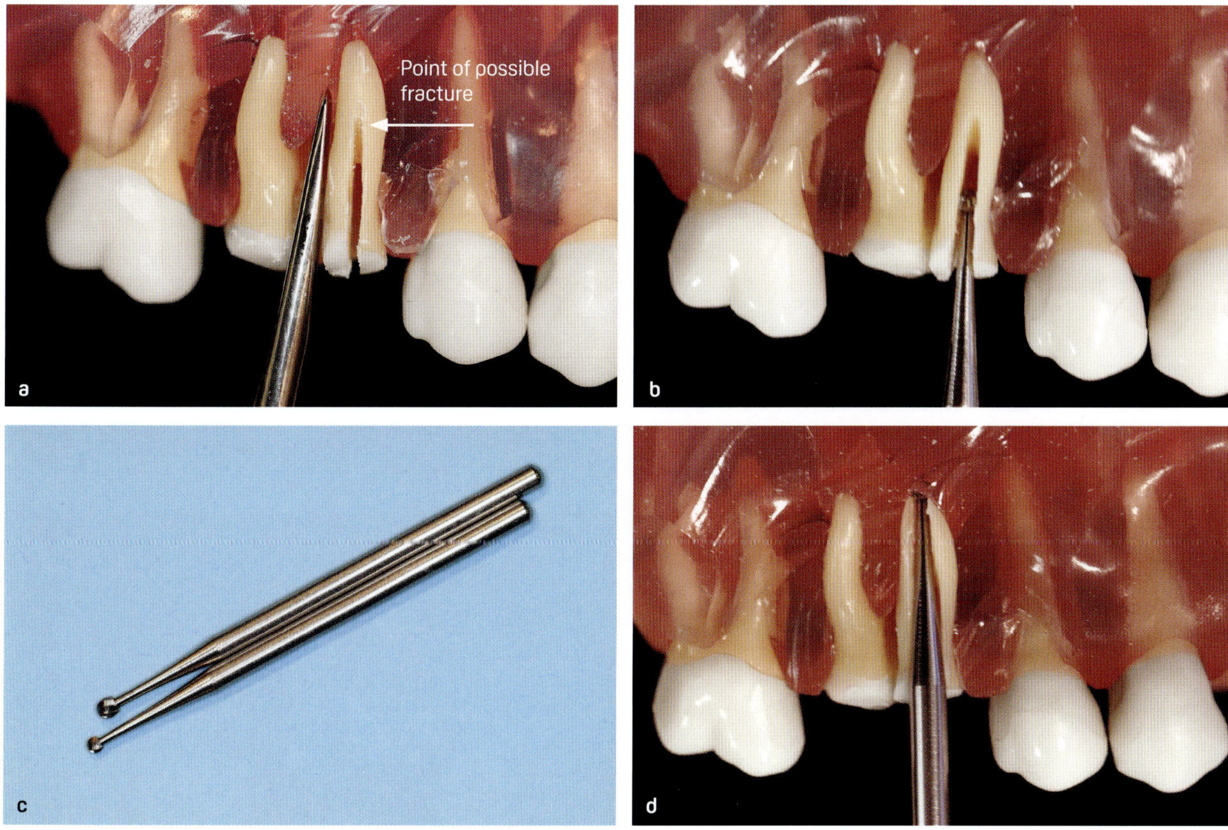

FIG 9-27 The mesiobuccal root of the maxillary right first molar is used as an example of a root requiring vertical sectioning. *(a)* Thin Directa Luxator L2S elevator pressuring the incompletely sectioned mesiobuccal root. There is a risk of fracturing the root at the depth of the cut, leaving the apex attached to the remaining root (gingiva removed for visualization purposes). *(b)* Root not sectioned entirely through apex. A wider opening is needed to allow room for the shank of the straight handpiece bur. *(c)* Straight handpiece burs #6 *(top)* and #4 *(bottom)*; the smaller bur (#4) is used for smaller roots, and #6 is used for larger roots. *(d)* Straight handpiece bur #4 sectioning completely past the apex into bone.

The mesiobuccal and distobuccal roots ideally should be sectioned in a buccopalatal direction so that mobilization of the root fragments does not damage the buccal bone. However, they can be sectioned in a mesiodistal direction if they are too thin to be sectioned in a buccopalatal direction. It is also preferable that the palatal roots are sectioned in a buccopalatal direction so that mobilization of the root fragments does not damage the palatal bone. However, they too can be sectioned in a mesiodistal direction, as long as care is taken to avoid damaging the palatal bone when pressuring the sectioned pieces.

It is very important to section all the way through the apex, since luxating two halves of incompletely sectioned roots may result in a fracture coronal to the apex, leaving the root tip connected to one of the sectioned root pieces (Fig 9-27a). If the surgical-length crosscut fissure bur does not reach the apex, use a straight handpiece bur #4 or #6 to completely cut through the apex. This requires opening up the cut wider at the coronal aspect to allow room for the shank of the straight handpiece bur (Figs 9-27b and 9-27c). When the root is completely sectioned through the apex, you will feel the bur drop into the softer bone (Fig 9-27d). Cut toward the palatal and buccal slightly to make sure the cut is through the entire root structure. Then, introduce an elevator between the root sections and, using gentle rotation, pressure them laterally (Fig 9-28). Try not to fracture the bone surrounding the roots. If pressuring between the roots does not mobilize them, then once again excise the periodontal ligament fibers around the roots with a thin periotome or ¼ round bur, attempting to cut more in the direction of the root, not the bone of the socket wall.

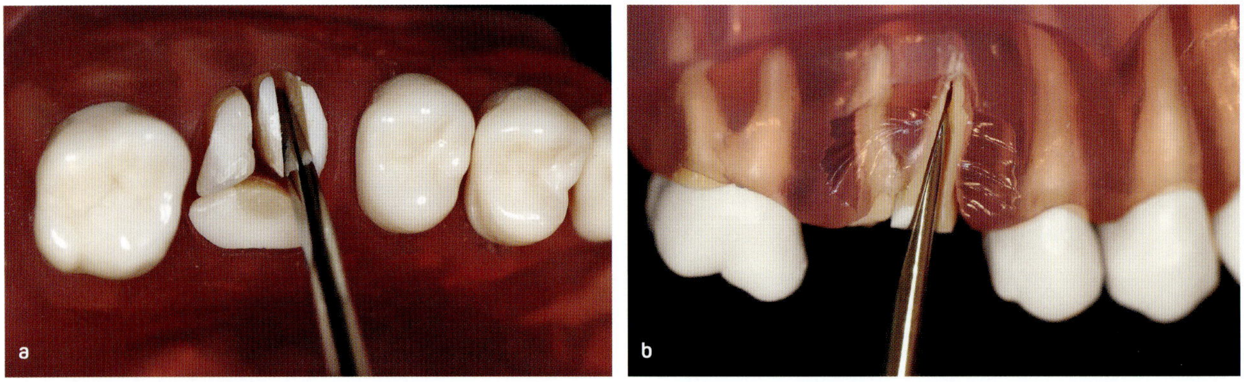

FIG 9-28 *(a and b)* Thin Directa Luxator L2S elevator used with a gentle twisting motion to pressure the maxillary right first molar mesiobuccal root halves mesially and distally.

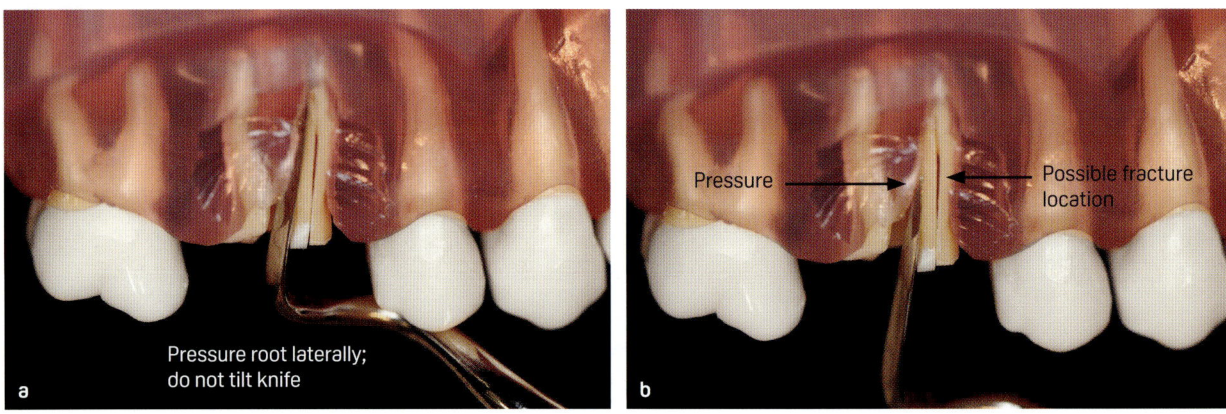

FIG 9-29 *(a)* Placement of Hu-Friedy Orban knife KO1/2IU as far apically as possible to pressure, rather than tilt, the sectioned mesiobuccal root half, reducing the risk of root fracture. *(b)* If the knife is positioned only halfway down the root surface, there is a greater chance the root will fracture as it is pressured into the space created by sectioning the root. Pressure on the coronal half of the sectioned root stresses the mid-root area, leading to possible fracture, even if it is fully sectioned through the apex.

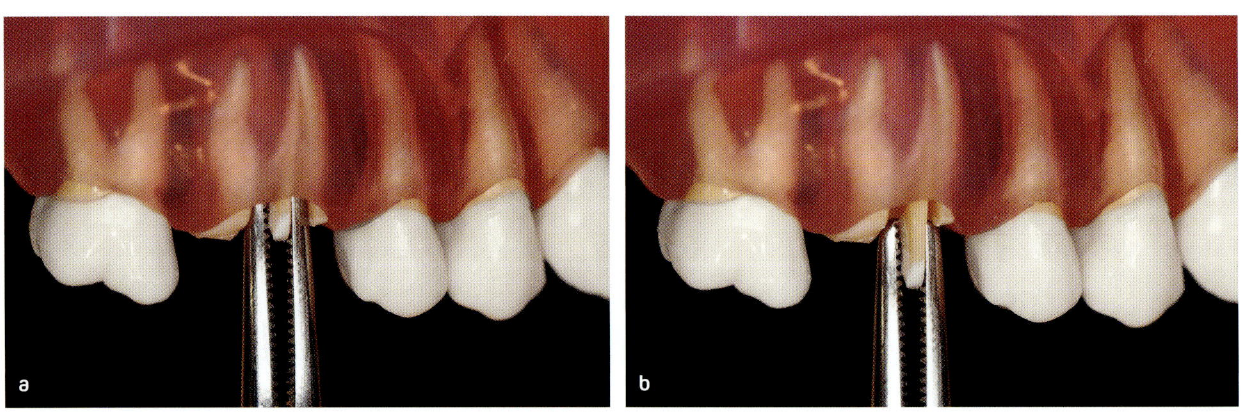

FIG 9-30 *(a and b)* Hemostat beaks are locked as far apically as possible on a mobile root section, which is removed with constant pulling pressure and a gentle back-and-forth motion.

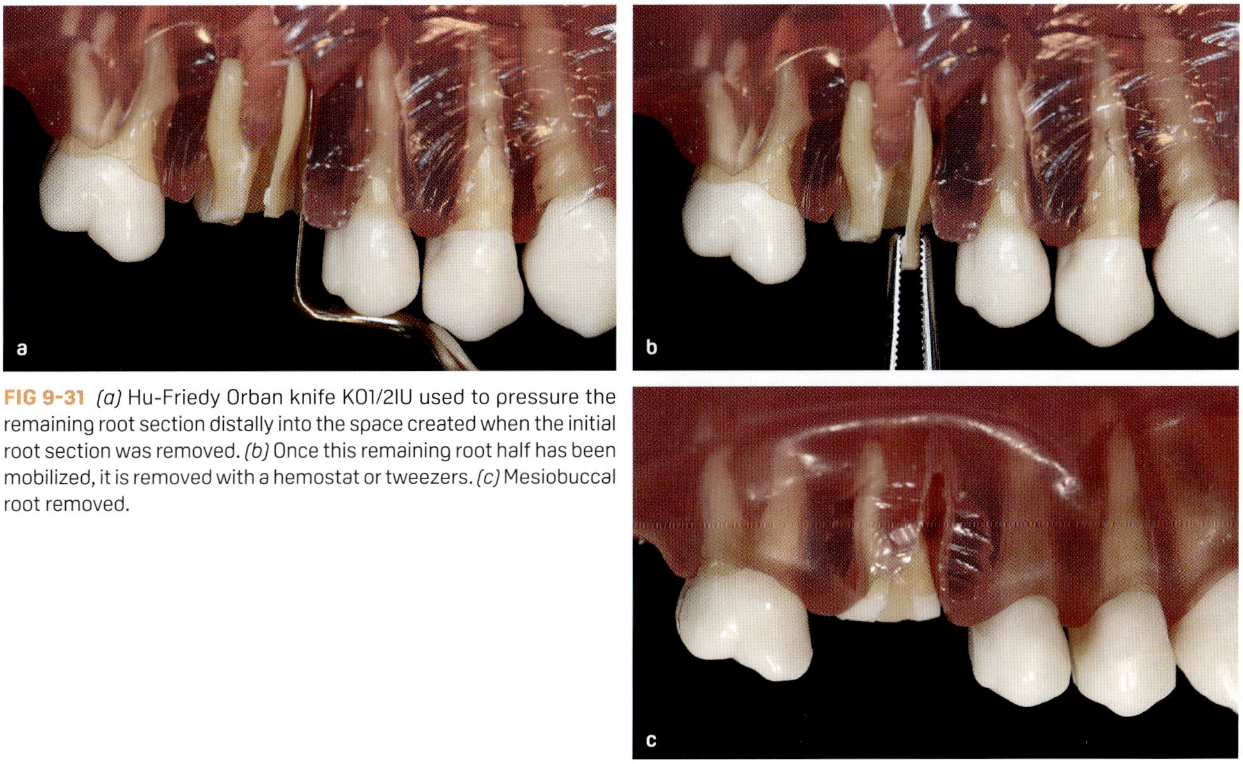

FIG 9-31 *(a)* Hu-Friedy Orban knife KO1/2IU used to pressure the remaining root section distally into the space created when the initial root section was removed. *(b)* Once this remaining root half has been mobilized, it is removed with a hemostat or tweezers. *(c)* Mesiobuccal root removed.

Enter Sulcus Laterally and Pressure Root Fragments into Sectioned Space

Enter the sulcus on the mesial and distal of the sectioned root with a thin elevator, Orban knife, or periotome and gently pressure the root fragments mesially and distally into the sectioned space. It is important to make sure the instrument is seated as far apically as possible into the sulcus before applying pressure. This gives you more leverage to push the entire root fragment laterally instead of tipping it, which may cause the root tip to fracture (Fig 9-29).

You may find that reentering the sectioned area and cutting deeper between the root fragments may be required. Be aware that you are pressuring against the adjacent bone, so do this in a gentle manner, paying attention to the thickness and density of the adjacent bone. The mesial and distal bone is usually thicker than the buccal and palatal bone and therefore is less vulnerable to damage from instrument pressure.

If this does not mobilize the root fragments, it may be necessary to section them again, this time in a mesiodistal direction, trying to avoid the mesial and distal socket walls as much as possible. This is more applicable to larger roots, but smaller roots may require this step, at which time you are actually drilling out most of the root. Again, it is necessary to drill through the apex; feeling the bur drop into softer bone is an indication that you are past the apex. Enter the sectioned space with a thin elevator and gently pressure the root fragments laterally. Then, pressure the sectioned fragments from the sulcus into the space created by sectioning the roots.

Once root segments are mobilized, lock onto an individual fragment with a hemostat or tweezers and use a gentle "wiggling" motion with constant pulling pressure to remove it from the socket (Fig 9-30). After one root section is removed, pressure the remaining root section with an Orban knife or thin elevator into the space created by removal of the first root section (Fig 9-31a). Then, remove this second root section (Figs 9-31b and 9-31c).

Once root removal is complete, proceed to socket debridement (see chapter 11).

Complications

If the root is not sectioned entirely through the apex or if the apex fractures, atraumatic removal is difficult. The following steps will help reduce the severity of such complications.

As mentioned earlier, if the root is not sectioned entirely through the apex, pressuring the root into the space may result in a horizontal fracture at the depth of the cut (see Fig 9-27a). If horizontal fracture occurs, remove the loose root fragment. The choice is then to attempt to pressure the remaining root, with the apex attached, into the space created by removing the root fragment or to section through the apex.

If the remaining root is pressured into the space created by removing the root fragment (RSCET; Fig 9-32), the risk is another horizontal root fracture, leaving the entire apex. This approach is more successful in softer maxillary bone. Attempting this in the denser mandibular bone will result in fractures more frequently. The other option is to section through the apex (Fig 9-33).

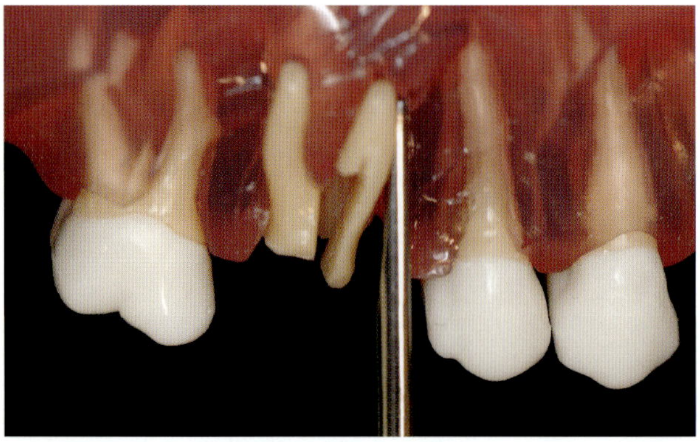

FIG 9-32 The thin Directa Luxator L2S elevator is used to pressure the remaining mesiobuccal root, with apex attached, into the space created by removing the root fragment (RSCET).

A fractured apex is a complication we will all experience. Sectioning entirely through the apex is necessary to help prevent these complications.

Once root removal is complete, proceed to socket debridement (see chapter 11).

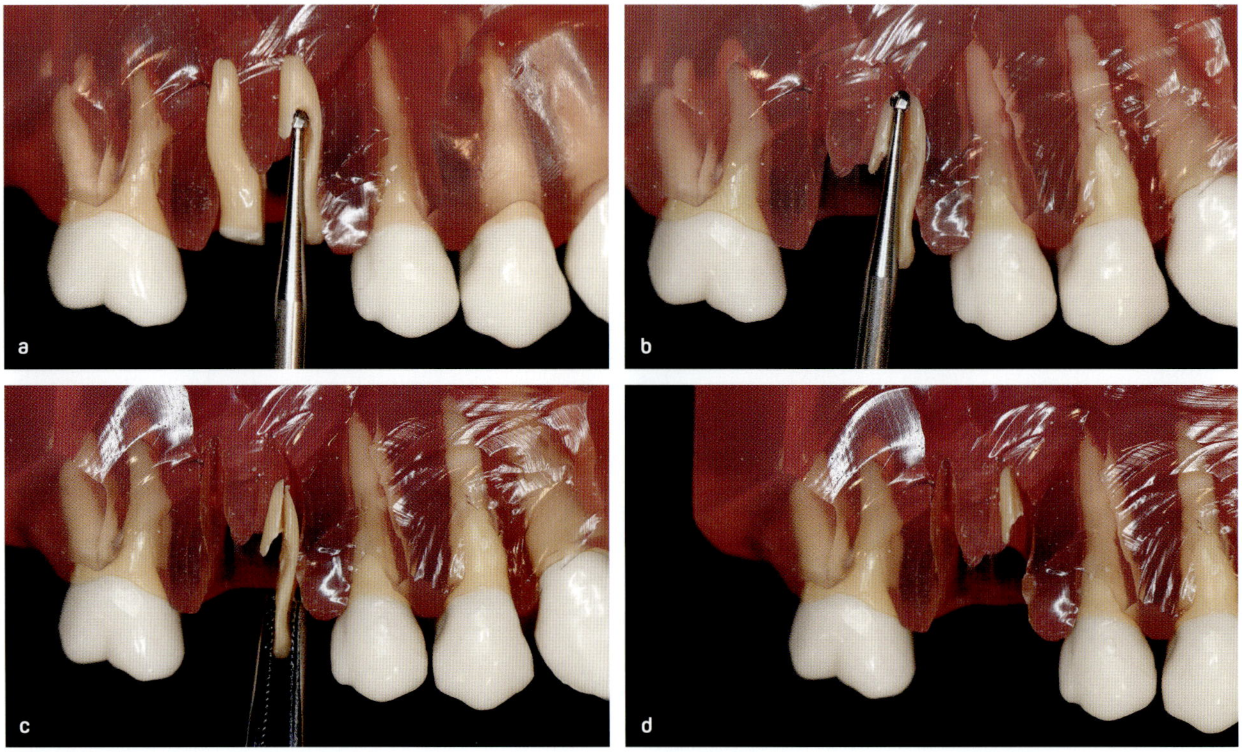

FIG 9-33 *(a and b)* If horizontal fracture occurs, remove the loose root fragment and use a straight handpiece bur #4 or #6 to completely section the root through the apex. Once through the apex, use an Orban knife to pressure the root half into the space created by removal of the root fragment. *(c)* Remove the long root fragment with tweezers. *(d)* Half apex remaining. This can be mobilized using a thin elevator and then removed with tweezers or by flushing with sterile saline.

10

Atraumatic Extraction of the Mandibular Molars: Divide and Divide Again, Then Conquer

The following atraumatic extraction techniques apply to mandibular molars with minimal to no mobility and good bone support. Obviously, teeth with Class II or III mobility can usually be removed atraumatically if there is adequate crown structure to grasp with a forceps. Also, it may not be necessary to use all of the following techniques to atraumatically remove a tooth. Some of the steps may be deemed nonproductive or not applicable to the clinical situation and therefore can be skipped at the discretion of the operating dentist.

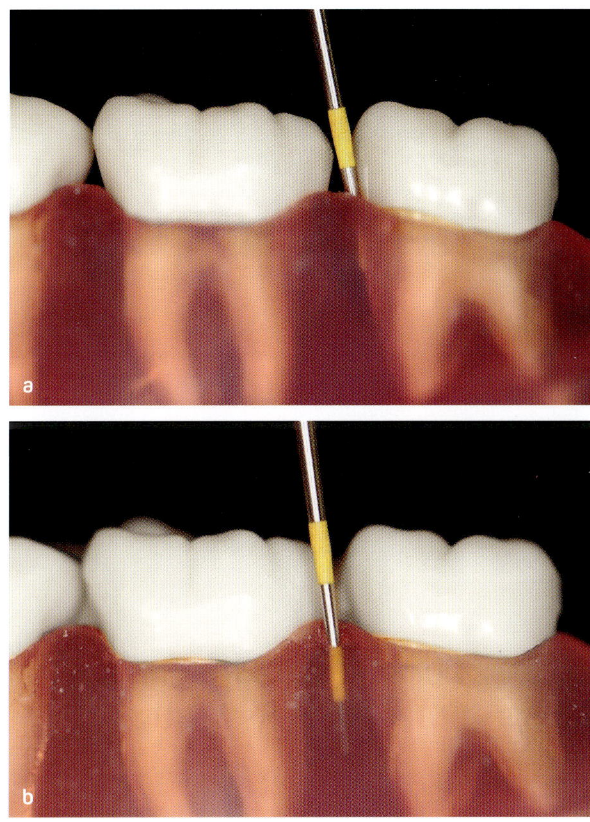

FIG 10-1 Verifying adequate anesthesia. *(a)* Probing the mesiobuccal sulcus of the mandibular left second molar. *(b)* Probing the gingiva between the mandibular left first and second molars.

Verify Profound Anesthesia

Probe the sulcus with a periodontal probe and stimulate the adjacent gingiva, especially on the lingual, to confirm you have profound anesthesia (Fig 10-1). If anesthesia is inadequate, administer either another nerve block or infiltration into the sulcus and adjacent gingiva circumferentially (Fig 10-2). For quickest onset, use 4% articaine with 1:100,000 epinephrine. For hemostasis, 2% lidocaine 1:100,000 epinephrine is helpful.

A bite block can be used to stabilize the mandible; this also helps patients hold their mouth open during the procedure, reducing muscle fatigue.

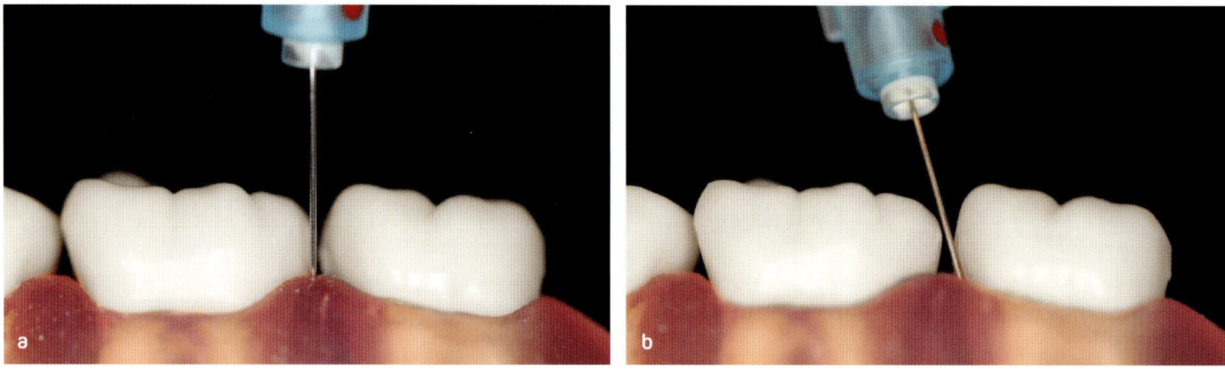

FIG 10-2 Supplementing anesthesia in adjacent gingiva and sulcus. *(a)* Infiltration directly into the buccal papilla between the mandibular left first and second molars. *(b)* Infiltration into the mesiobuccal sulcus of the mandibular left second molar.

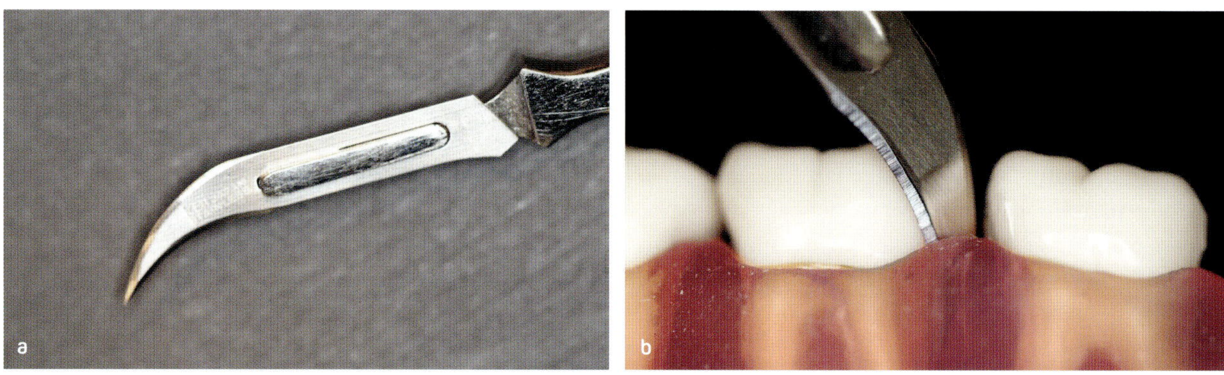

FIG 10-3 *(a)* A 12D scalpel blade. *(b)* The scalpel blade inserted into the distobuccal sulcus of the mandibular left first molar to release the periodontal ligament fibers using a back-and-forth rocking motion with vertical pressure.

Release Periodontal Ligament Fibers Without Flap Reflection

Note that some practitioners remove the crown as the first step. They feel that getting the crown out of the way and just dealing with the root(s) is the most efficient and atraumatic method to remove a tooth. For the purposes of this chapter, we will assume the crown will be left in place for these initial procedures.

Using a 12D scalpel blade, enter the sulcus on the mesial, distal, and lingual, but not the buccal due to the thin buccal bone being vulnerable to resorption and fracture. Apply vertical pressure with a back-and-forth rocking motion (Fig 10-3).

Optional procedure

Use a periotome to excise the periodontal ligament as deeply as possible two times in the mesial, distal, and lingual sulci (Fig 10-4). Avoid the buccal, where the bone is thin. Use a back-and-forth motion with vertical pressure. However, it may be difficult to get into the periodontal ligament space due to lack of space or ankylosis. If that is the case, proceed to the recommended procedure below.

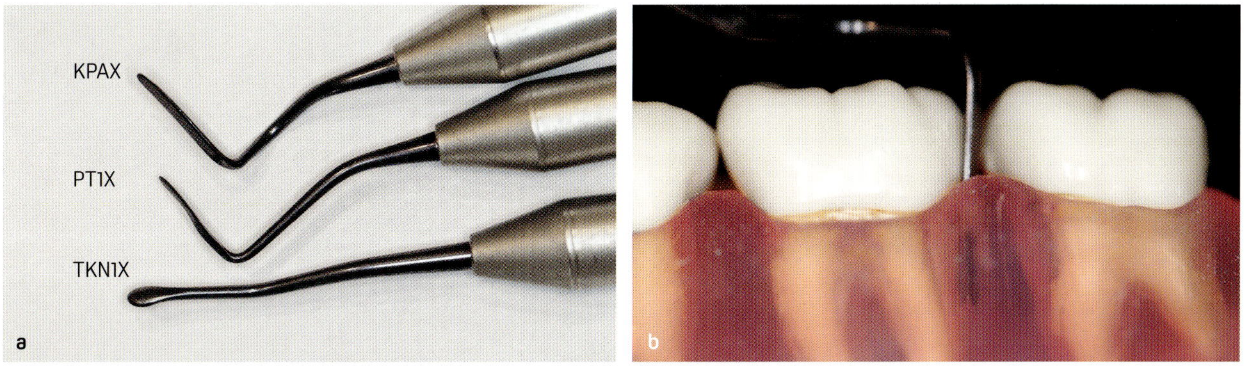

FIG 10-4 *(a)* Hu-Friedy periotomes. *(b)* Periotome inserted into the distobuccal sulcus of the mandibular left first molar to excise periodontal ligament fibers. Use vertical pressure and a back-and-forth rocking motion. Avoid the thin buccal bone.

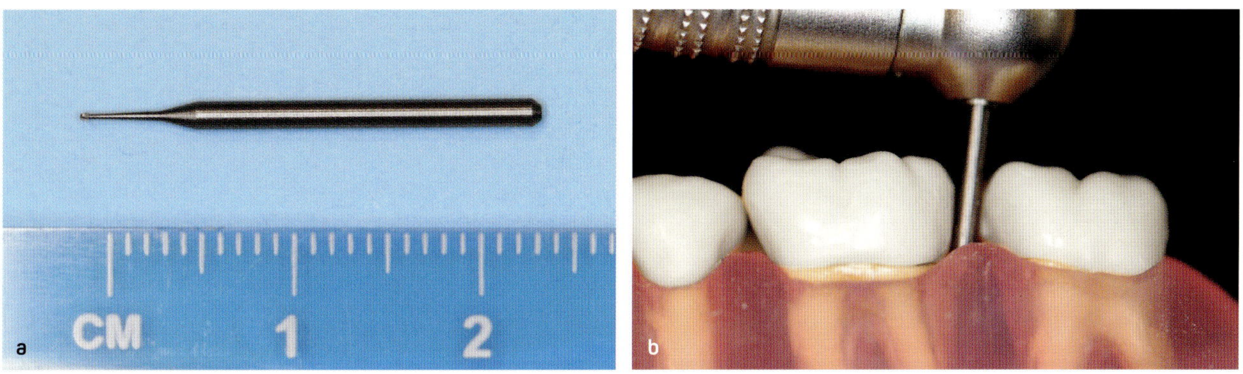

FIG 10-5 *(a)* Surgical-length high-speed ¼ round bur used to separate the root from the bone in the sulcus. *(b)* The bur is inserted in the distobuccal sulcus of the mandibular left first molar with an up-and-down pumping motion and light pressure against the root, not the bone.

Recommended procedure

Use a surgical-length high-speed ¼ round bur to further sever the periodontal ligament fibers (Fig 10-5a). Use an up-and-down pumping motion in the periodontal ligament space at the mesial, distal, and palatal, but avoid the buccal since the thin buccal bone is vulnerable to resorption and fracture (Fig 10-5b). Extend as far apically as possible, gently pressuring in the direction of the tooth root rather than the bone of the socket wall. This opening of the periodontal ligament space releases the tooth from the adjacent bone, making it easier to remove, and creates space for a thin elevator to enter and pressure the root.

A periotome, scalpel, or round bur may be used in any order.

Attempt Tooth Movement Coronally Without Flap Reflection

Introduce a thin elevator (Fig 10-6) at the mesiobuccal and distobuccal and, using a twisting motion, attempt to move the tooth coronally (Fig 10-7).

If there is adequate crown structure present for luxation of any kind, the following will be helpful.

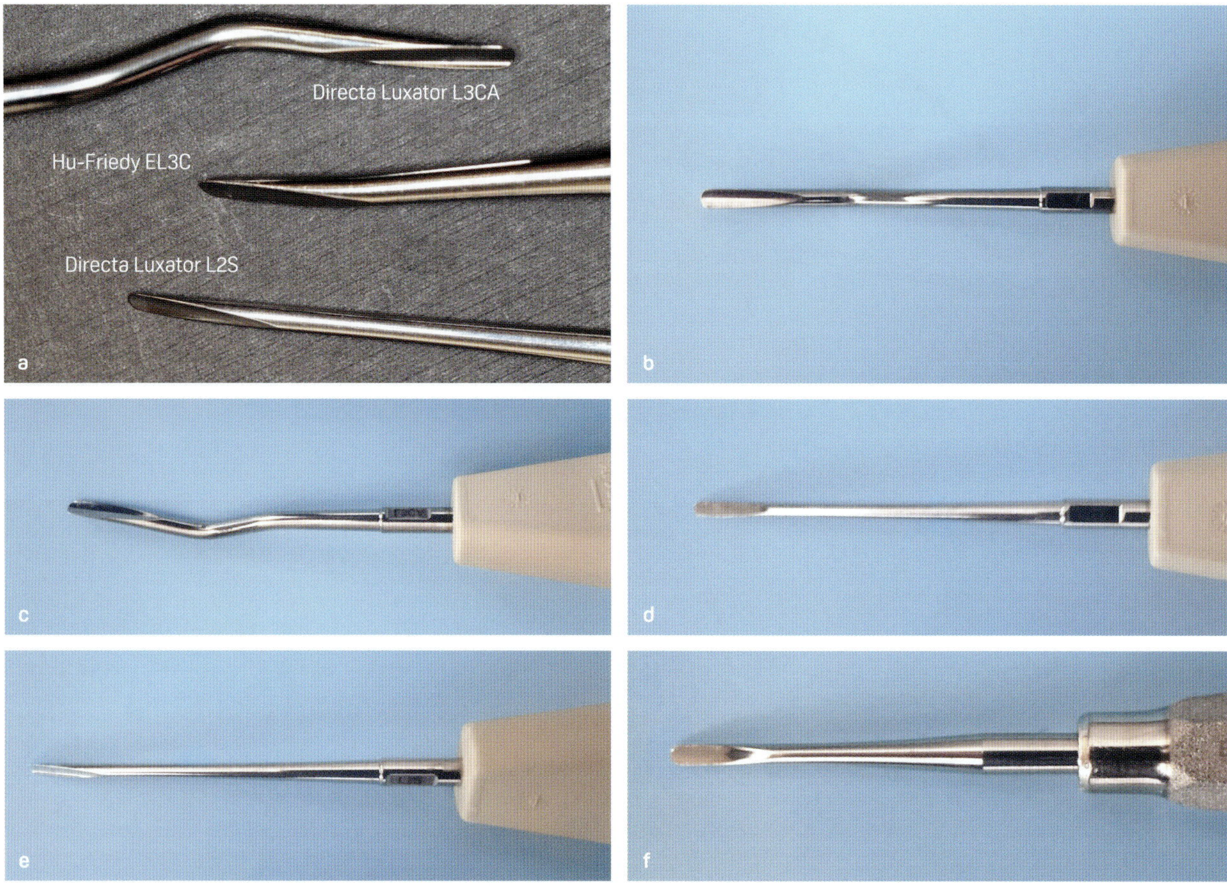

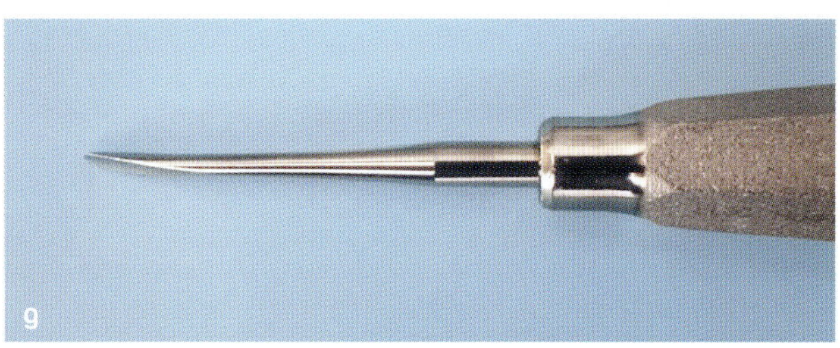

FIG 10-6 *(a)* Examples of thin elevators. *(b)* Directa Luxator L3CA top view. *(c)* Directa Luxator L3CA side view. *(d)* Directa Luxator L2S top view. *(e)* Directa Luxator L2S side view. *(f)* Hu-Friedy EL3C top view. *(g)* Hu-Friedy EL3C side view.

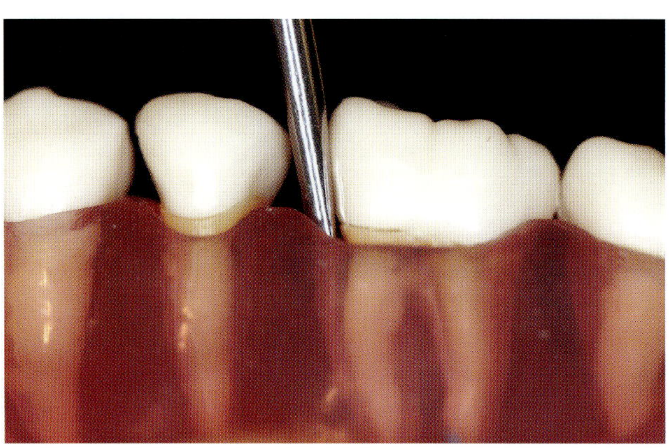

FIG 10-7 Directa Luxator L2S elevator inserted in the mesial sulcus of the mandibular left first molar.

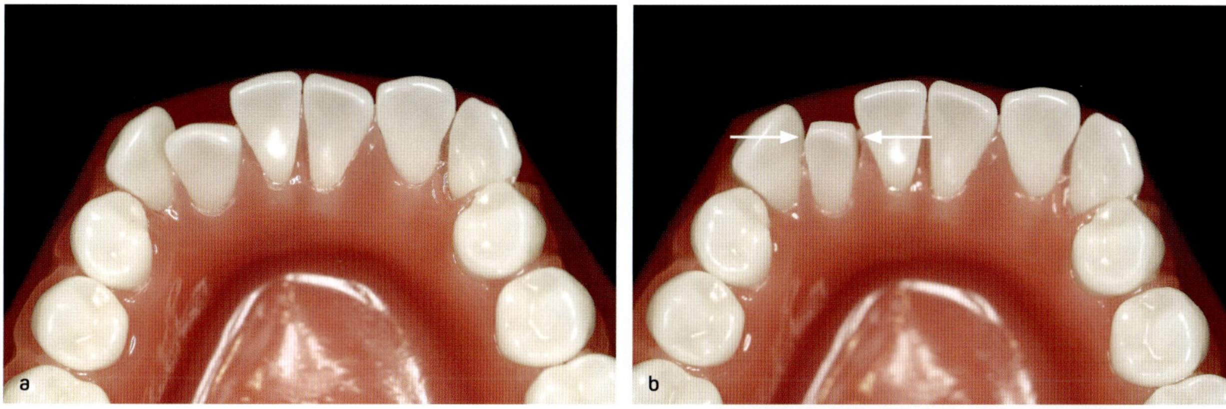

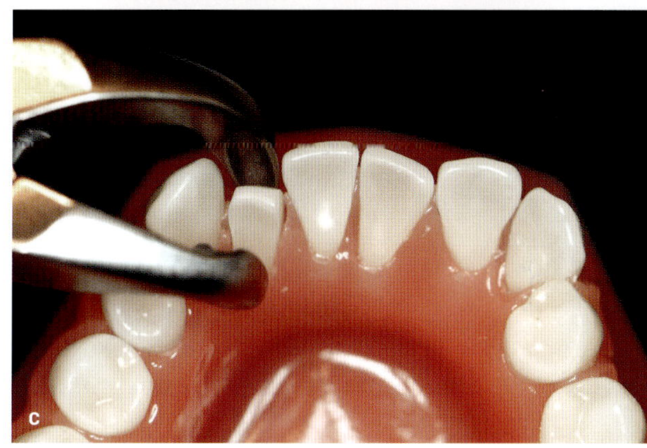

FIG 10-8 *(a)* Mandibular left lateral incisor overlapped with the adjacent canine and central incisor. Rotating the lateral incisor with a forceps will apply pressure to (and may cause increased mobility of) these adjacent teeth. *(b)* The mesial and distal contacts of the lateral incisor have been reduced. *(c)* Now rotation of the lateral incisor with a forceps will be less harmful to adjacent teeth.

Reduce Interproximal Contacts

We are attempting to remove a tooth as atraumatically as possible, and this pertains not only to the tooth being extracted but also to the adjacent teeth, their restorations, and the rest of the mouth as well. If we were to luxate a tooth with tight or overlapping contacts, we would be pressuring the adjacent contacts and therefore moving the adjacent teeth. (If multiple adjacent teeth are being removed, this concept does not apply; luxation of a tooth with tight or overlapping contacts may actually help loosen adjacent teeth planned for extraction.) Therefore, where teeth are overlapped or crowded, I feel it is important to reduce the interproximal contacts on a single tooth to be removed. Note that if interproximal contacts are present, but luxation does not move or harm adjacent teeth or restorations, then reduction of interproximal contacts is not necessary. If contacts are overlapping on one side only, rotate the tooth in the direction that does not increase contact pressure. Figure 10-8 presents overlapping mandibular incisors as an example.

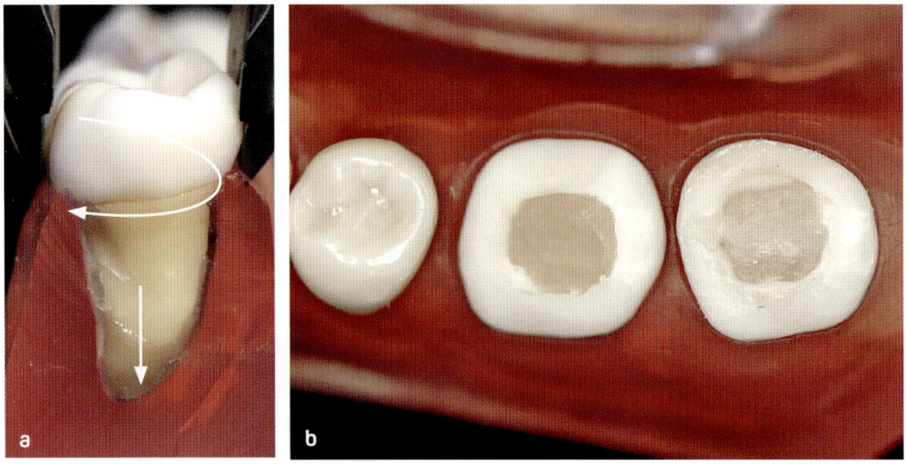

FIG 10-9 *(a)* Forceps applied as far apically as possible without damaging bone or soft tissue. First apply vertical pressure, then rotational movement. *(b)* Crowns removed to show trapezoidal shape of mandibular molars. Excessive rotation may fracture the socket wall or roots.

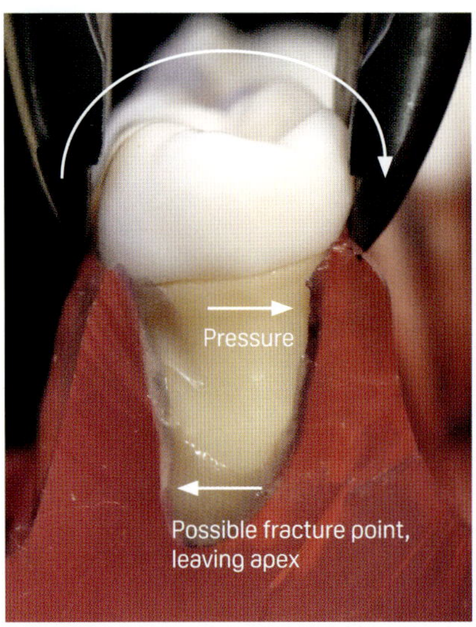

FIG 10-10 Pressure applied coronally with forceps toward the lingual of the mandibular left first molar, which also pressures the buccal surfaces of the mesial and distal roots. This may result in fracture of the apices.

Luxate Gently with Forceps

If the crown is intact and the roots are fused, forceps can be used to gently luxate and attempt removal of the tooth; however, because the roots are at different angles, this may damage the surrounding bone, so caution is recommended.

Engage the root surface apical to any restoration margins with mandibular molar forceps. Gently apply pressure apically and hold for 30 seconds. While continuing to apply apical pressure, gently luxate in a buccal and lingual direction with slight rotation to test the mobility of the tooth (Fig 10-9a). The reason for applying apical pressure while luxating is that it shifts the axis of rotation in an apical direction, reducing the chance for root fracture. Remember that the mandibular molars are trapezoidal in shape (Fig 10-9b); therefore, unless they have Class II or III mobility, it is recommended to avoid excessive rotation since this will expand the socket and may fracture the socket wall or roots.

If the bone on the buccal or palatal alveolar crest is especially thick, pressure can be placed in that direction. However, it is important to realize that when applying pressure coronally in a lateral direction toward the alveolar crest, the apical portion of the tooth will be forced against the opposite socket walls. This pressure can lead to fracture of one or more root apices, which would have to be retrieved (Fig 10-10). Mandibular bone is denser than maxillary bone; therefore, root fracture is more probable in the mandible, depending on the root anatomy.

If there is a full-coverage restoration, luxation may or may not remove the crown. If gentle luxation is not successful in removing the tooth, the crown (whether a cemented full-coverage restoration or natural tooth) should be sectioned horizontally about 1 mm coronal to the gingival margin as described in the next section.

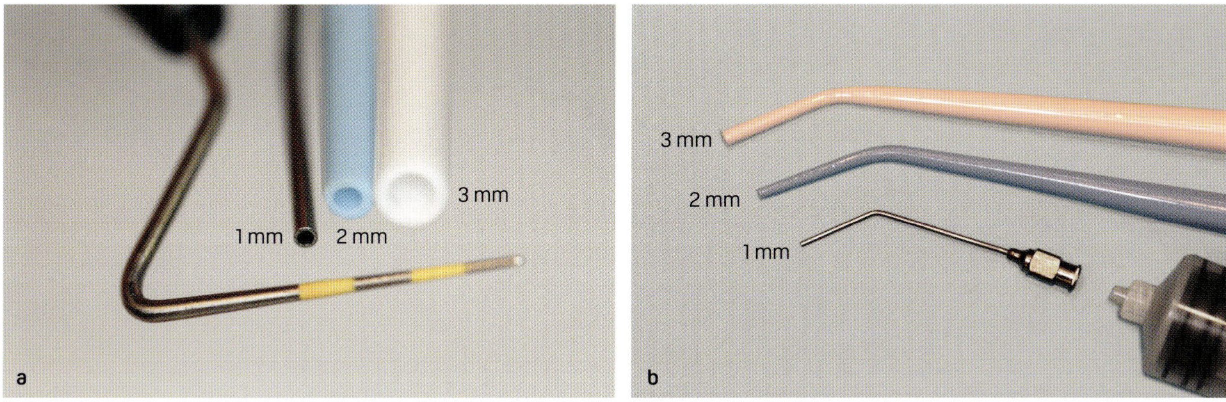

FIG 10-11 *(a and b)* Thin 1-mm irrigation tip and 2- and 3-mm-diameter suction tips used during sectioning of a crown.

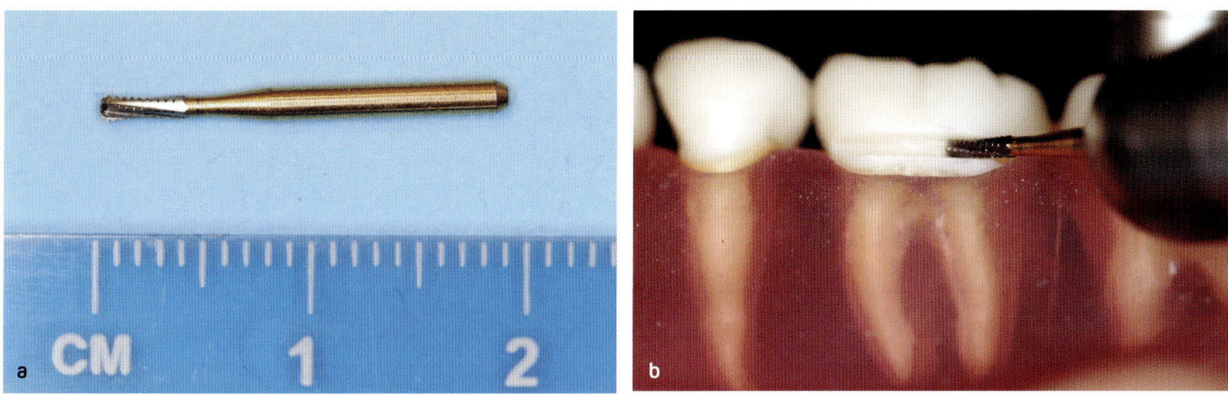

FIG 10-12 *(a)* Great White high-speed crosscut fissure bur used to horizontally section the crown. *(b)* Sectioning the mandibular left first molar crown 1 mm coronal to the free gingival margin.

Section Crown Horizontally at the Cementoenamel Junction

This technique can be used for mandibular molars with fused or non-fused roots. Some practitioners go right to this step for every extraction, feeling that it is the most efficient and atraumatic method.

When sectioning a crown or roots, it is important to use plenty of saline irrigation with a thin irrigation tip to remove tooth debris and to use a thin suction tip to suction within the drill cuts and sockets. This allows you to see and feel in these areas (Fig 10-11). Section the crown 1 mm coronal to the gingival margin using a Great White (SS White) high-speed crosscut fissure bur (Fig 10-12). It is important to be aware of the gingival margin location to avoid lacerating the gingiva. Leaving the root 1 mm above the gingival margin allows a starting point for a thin elevator, surgical-length ¼ round bur, or periotome to enter the sulcus to pressure the root.

Obviously, it's much easier to section through tooth structure or a composite restoration as compared to a metal restoration. Regardless of the material, section two-thirds of the way through the crown, and then, using an elevator, gently pry off the crown. Using a football-shaped high-speed diamond bur, smooth the remaining tooth structure to a fairly flat surface approximately 1 mm coronal to the gingival margin (Fig 10-13).

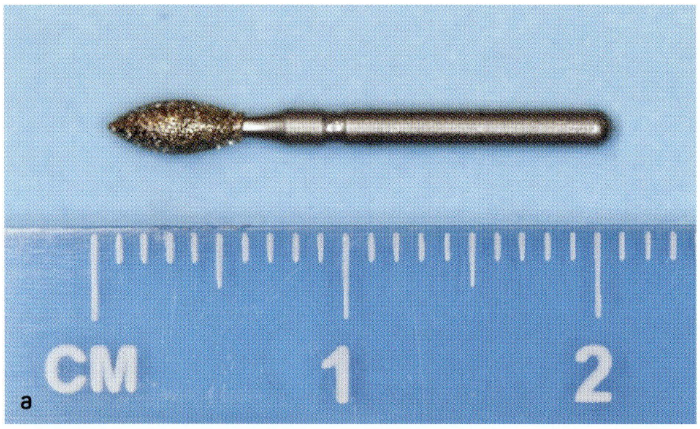

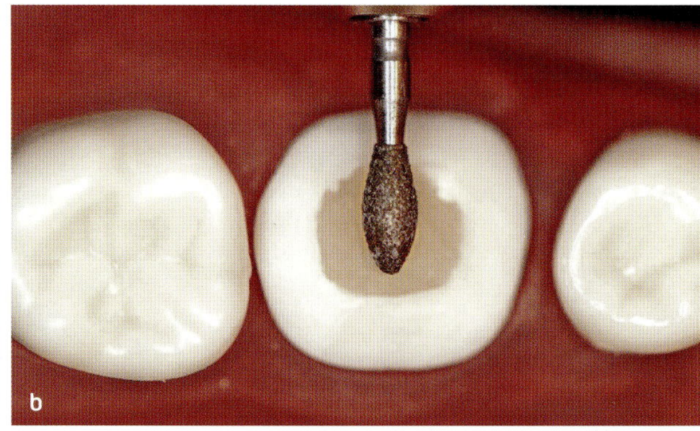

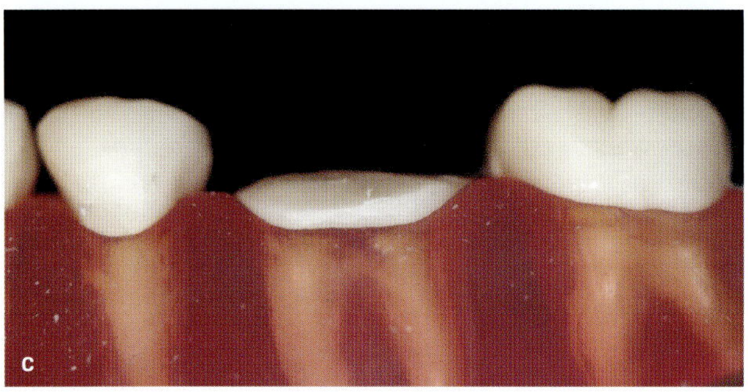

FIG 10-13 *(a)* High-speed football diamond bur used to smooth the remaining root to a level 1 mm above the gingival margin after sectioning off the crown. *(b)* Bur used to smooth the remaining root of the mandibular left first molar. *(c)* Buccal view of the mandibular left first molar sectioned 1 mm above the gingival margin.

Removing the crown allows you to see the remaining root structure, including where the roots divide, and to determine the best location to section vertically. Vertical fractures may be evident also. A dye such as To Dye For (Roydent) may be used to help visualize possible fractures.

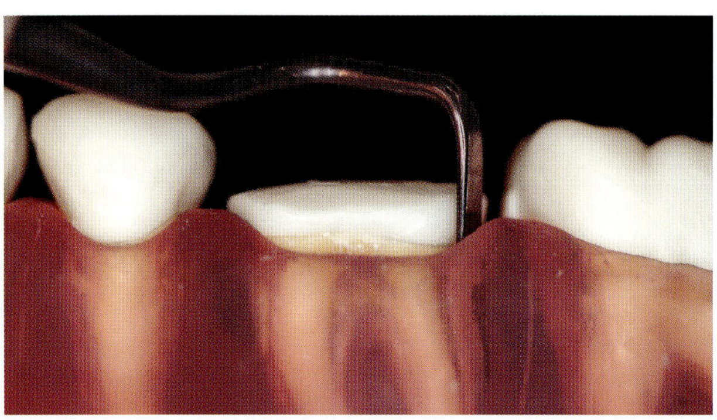

FIG 10-14 Periotome in the distal sulcus of the mandibular left first molar using vertical pressure and a back-and-forth rocking motion. Avoid the buccal, where bone is thin.

Optional procedure

Release the periodontal ligament fibers again using a narrow periotome (see Fig 10-4a). Enter the sulcus on the lingual, mesial, and distal, applying vertical pressure and a back-and-forth rocking motion to excise the periodontal ligament fibers further apically (Fig 10-14).

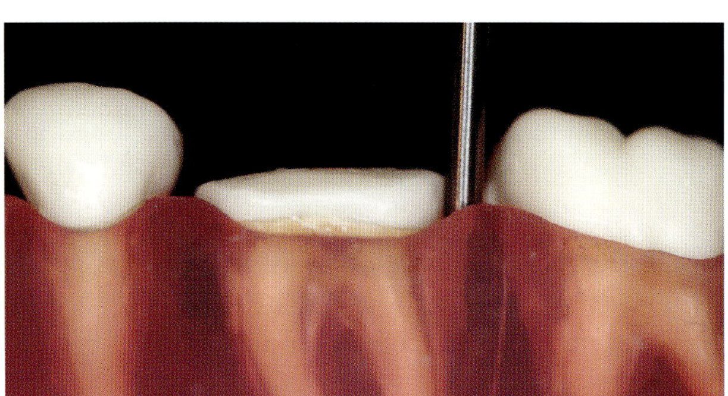

FIG 10-15 Surgical-length high-speed ¼ round bur used with a gentle up-and-down motion in the distobuccal sulcus of the mandibular left first molar, exerting pressure toward the root, not the bone of the socket wall.

Recommended procedure

Instead of a periotome, you can use a surgical-length high-speed ¼ round bur to further sever the periodontal ligament fibers (Fig 10-15). Attempt to cut more in the direction of the root rather than the bone of the socket wall. Excising periodontal ligament fibers like this detaches the root from the bone, allowing for easier extraction. Avoid the buccal aspect because bone in this area is thin.

Use Thin Elevator to Mobilize Tooth Without Flap Reflection

Introducing a thin elevator (see Fig 10-6a) at the mesial and distal, use a twisting motion to attempt to move the tooth coronally (Fig 10-16). This is done to begin mobilizing the tooth. The most atraumatic technique for removing a mandibular molar is to separate the roots since each root draws in a different direction.

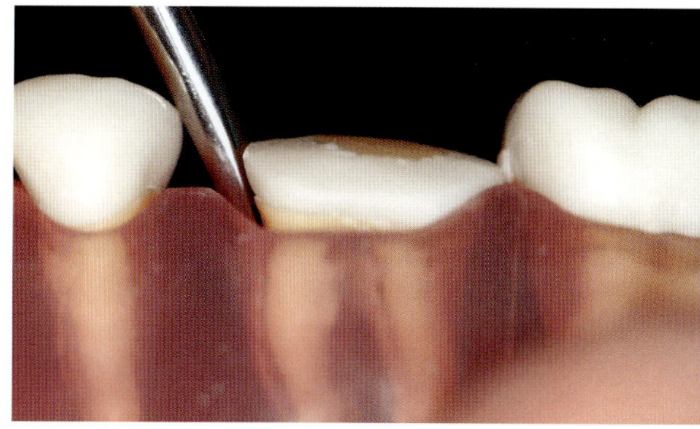

FIG 10-16 A thin elevator is used to gently luxate the tooth with a twisting motion, attempting to mobilize it.

Section Vertically Between Roots

Multirooted mandibular teeth usually require sectioning buccolingually between the roots since there are two separate roots that draw in different directions. If an attempt is made to remove the tooth in one piece, one or more of the roots may fracture and bone may be damaged in the process. Some mandibular second and third molars have fused roots, but even in these cases, the roots are much easier to remove if they are separated from each other.

Evaluate the radiographic appearance of the roots to determine the depth of cut required to separate them. Use a surgical-length high-speed crosscut fissure bur to section in a buccolingual direction between the mesial and distal roots (Fig 10-17). Be careful to cut only tooth structure and to minimize bone damage as much as possible.

This technique is termed the *root space creation extraction technique* (*RSCET*). The concept involves using a bur to remove tooth structure and creating a space into which the divided roots can be pressured, away from the sulcus and socket wall. In this way, tooth roots can be removed without removing supporting bone. It is important that you have thin sterile saline irrigation and suction tips that reach the apices of the roots you are sectioning, allowing you to irrigate and suction the drill cuts, removing tooth debris for visualization.

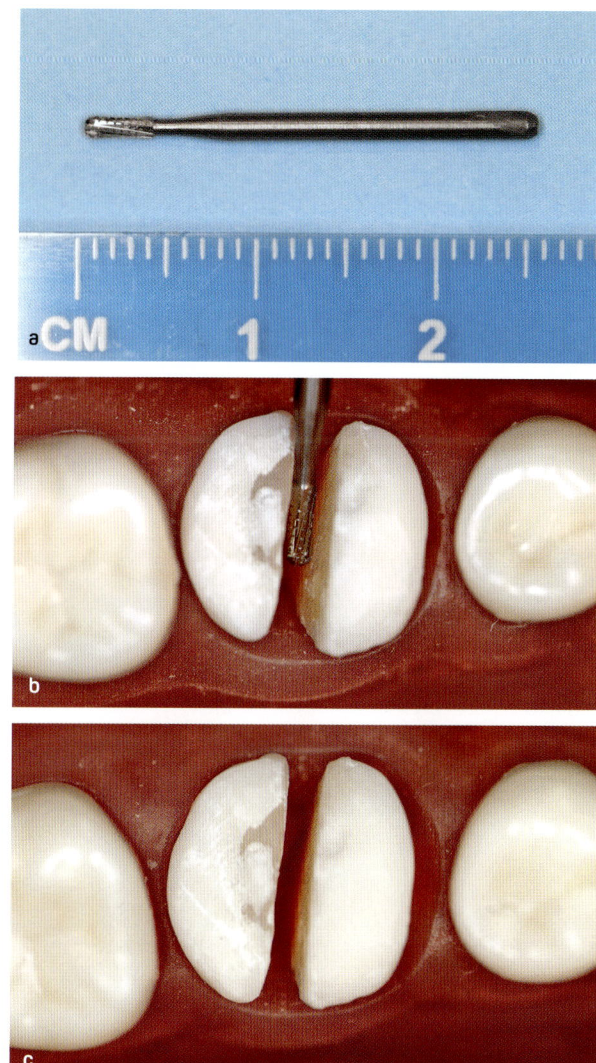

FIG 10-17 *(a)* Surgical-length high-speed crosscut fissure bur. *(b and c)* The bur is used to section vertically and buccolingually in the furcation between the mesial and distal roots of the mandibular left first molar.

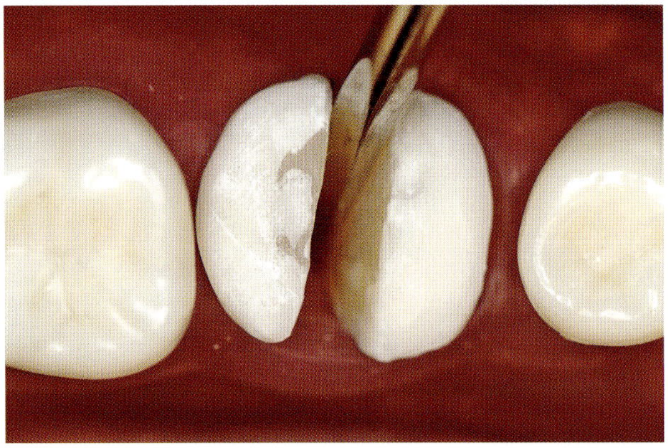

FIG 10-18 Thin Hu-Friedy EL3C elevator used with a gentle twisting motion to separate and mobilize the mandibular left first molar roots.

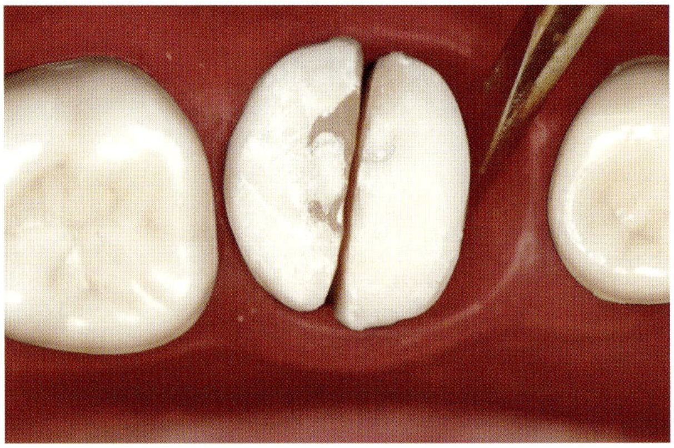

FIG 10-19 Gently pressuring the mesial root distally with a thin Hu-Friedy EL3C elevator.

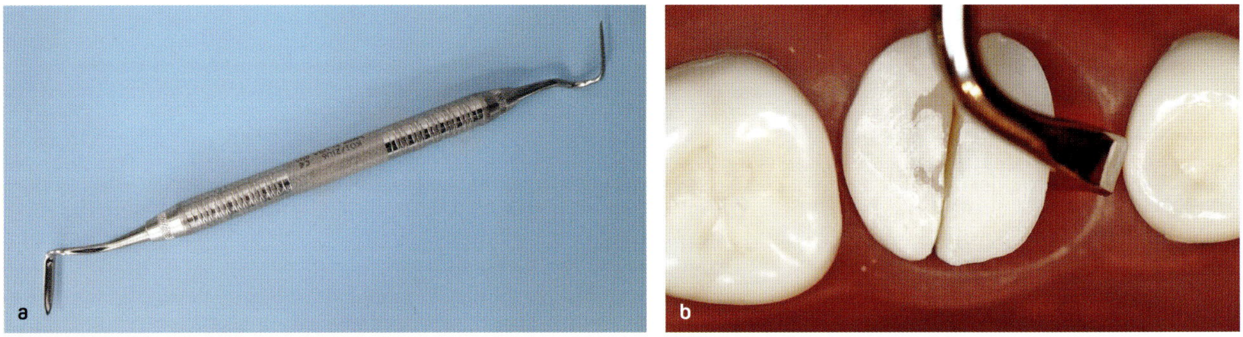

FIG 10-20 *(a)* Hu-Friedy Orban knife KO1/2IU. *(b)* Using the Orban knife to pressure the mesial root distally into the space created by sectioning the roots. It is important to insert the instrument as deeply as possible into the periodontal ligament space before pressuring. This helps prevent fracturing of the root.

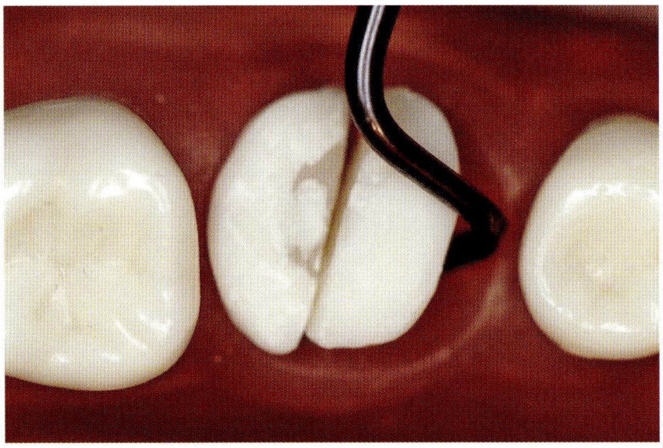

FIG 10-21 Using a periotome to pressure the mesial root distally into the space created by sectioning the roots.

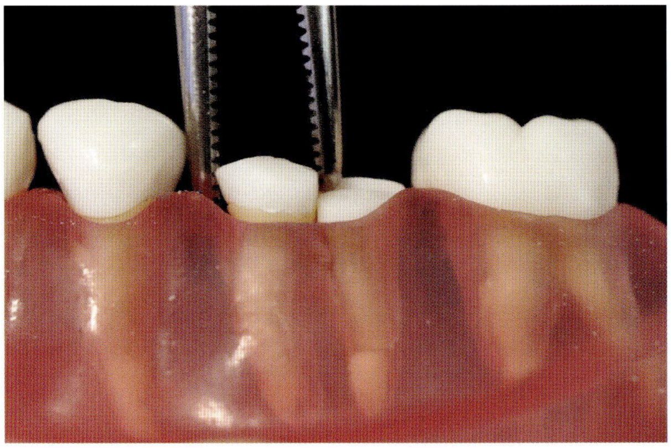

FIG 10-22 Hemostat locked onto the mesial root of the mandibular left first molar, using a back-and-forth motion and constant pulling pressure to mobilize and remove it from the socket.

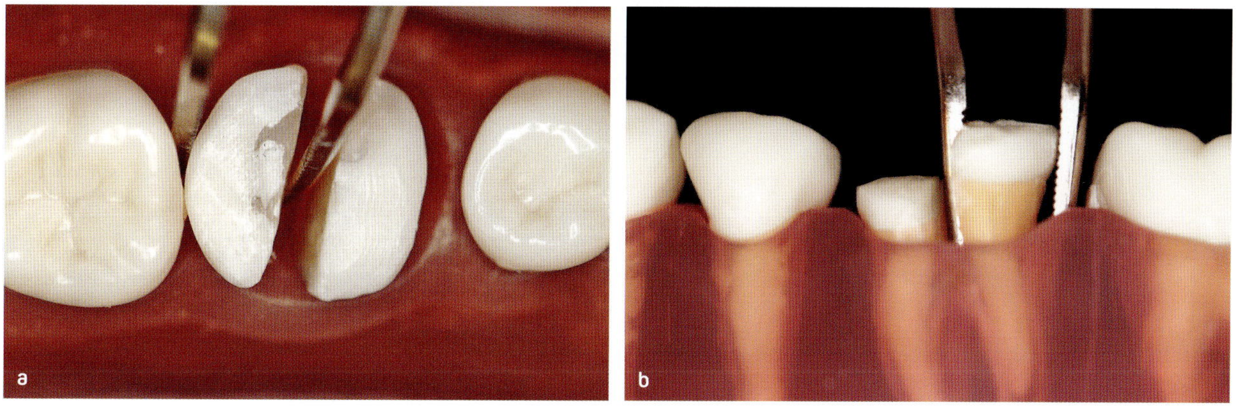

FIG 10-23 *(a and b)* Tweezers used to remove the mobile distal root of the mandibular left first molar.

Elevate Gently Between Roots

Introduce an elevator between the sectioned roots and, using a gentle twisting motion, pressure the roots laterally (Fig 10-18). Be aware that you are also pressuring the bone laterally, so if it looks like there is a weak area, avoid pressuring that area.

If pressuring between the roots does not mobilize them, use a periotome or surgical-length high-speed ¼ round bur to further excise the periodontal ligament fibers in the sulcus from the surfaces of the roots. Cut more in the direction of the root, not the bone of the socket wall.

Enter Sulcus Laterally and Pressure Roots into Sectioned Space

Insert a thin elevator, Hu-Friedy Orban knife KO1/2IU, or periotome mesial to the mesial root or distal to the distal root and pressure the root into the space created by sectioning the roots (Figs 10-19 to 10-21). It is important to insert the instrument as far apically as possible and to pressure the root laterally, not tilting the instrument, which could cause the root tip to fracture. Mandibular bone is much denser than maxillary bone; therefore, root fracture is more probable in the mandible.

If pressuring the roots into the space created by sectioning them does not mobilize them, excise the periodontal ligament fibers around the roots once again with a thin periotome or surgical length ¼ round bur. As before, attempt to cut more in the direction of the root, not the socket wall. You can also reenter the space between the roots with the surgical-length high-speed crosscut fissure bur and cut more in a buccolingual direction.

Once they are mobilized, the individual roots can be removed with a hemostat or tweezers. Lock the hemostat or tweezers onto a mobile root as far apically as possible and use a gentle back-and-forth motion with constant pulling pressure to remove the root from the socket (Figs 10-22 and 10-23). This technique is helpful in many instances where a tooth fragment has been mobilized and needs to be removed.

Another option is to use the Easy X-Trac System (A. Titan) or Benex Root Extraction System (Meisinger) (see chapter 12). For mandibular molars, the distal root is the only root large enough to be removed with these systems, both of which involve drilling a hole down the middle of the root canal space and inserting a threaded rod. This rod is pulled coronally with a wedging device, removing the root in one piece. Since the root is tapered, there is minimal trauma when it is removed in a vertical direction with the Easy X-Trac or Benex.

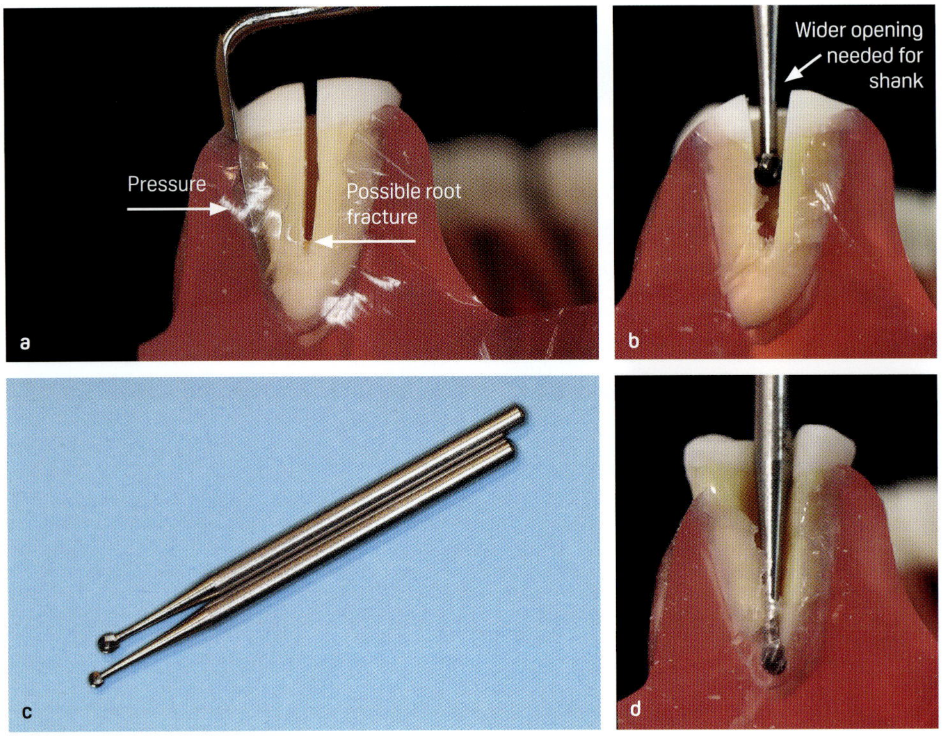

FIG 10-24 The distal root of the mandibular left first molar is used as an example of a root requiring vertical sectioning. *(a)* Orban knife pressuring at the buccal of the incompletely sectioned distal root. There is a risk of fracturing the root at the depth of the cut, leaving the apex attached to the remaining root (gingiva removed for visualization purposes). *(b)* Root not sectioned entirely through apex. A wider opening is needed to allow room for the shank of the straight handpiece bur. *(c)* Straight handpiece burs #6 *(top)* and #4 *(bottom)*; the smaller bur (#4) is used for smaller roots, and #6 is used for larger roots. *(d)* Straight handpiece bur #4 sectioning completely past the apex into bone.

Section Roots Themselves; Elevate Gently Between Root Fragments

If elevation and removal of the individual roots is not successful, then sectioning of the roots themselves is indicated. As before, use thin irrigation and suction tips that reach the apex of the roots you are sectioning to irrigate and suction the drill cuts.

The mesial and distal roots usually are sectioned in a mesiodistal direction since they are generally thin mesiodistally, making buccolingual sectioning difficult. It is very important to section all the way through the apex, since luxating two halves of an incompletely sectioned root may result in a fracture coronal to the apex, leaving the root tip connected to one of the sectioned root pieces (Fig 10-24a). If the surgical-length crosscut fissure bur does not reach the apex, use a straight handpiece bur #4 or #6 to completely cut through the apex. This requires opening up the cut wider at the coronal aspect to allow room for the shank of the straight handpiece bur (Figs 10-24b and 10-24c). Note that access may be difficult in the mandibular molar region with a straight handpiece. When the root is completely sectioned through the apex, you will feel the bur drop into the softer bone (Fig 10-24d). Cut toward the mesial and distal slightly to make sure the cut is entirely through the root structure. Then, introduce an elevator between the root sections and, using gentle rotation, pressure them buccally and lingually (Fig 10-25). Try not to fracture the bone surrounding the roots. If pressuring between the roots does not mobilize them, then once again excise the periodontal ligament fibers around the roots with a thin periotome or surgical-length high-speed ¼ round bur, attempting to cut more in the direction of the root, not the bone of the socket wall.

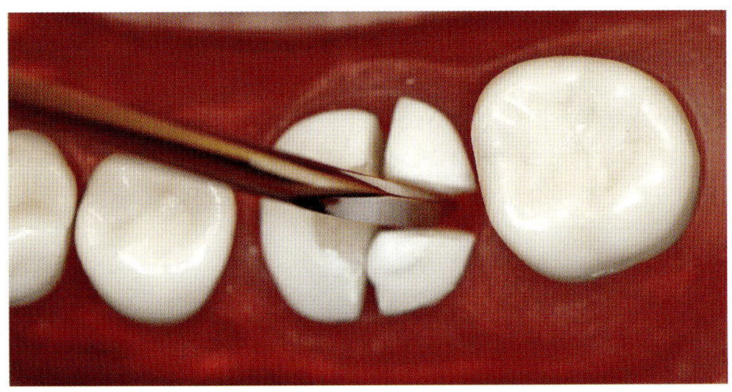

FIG 10-25 Thin Directa Luxator L2S elevator used with a gentle twisting motion to pressure the mandibular left first molar distal root halves buccally and lingually.

Enter Sulcus Buccally or Lingually and Pressure Root Fragments into Sectioned Space

Enter the sulcus on the buccal and lingual of the sectioned root with a thin elevator or Orban knife and gently pressure the root fragments buccally and lingually into the sectioned space. Be aware that you are also pressuring the bone buccally and lingually, so avoid pressuring any weak areas. When placing the thin elevator or Orban knife in the sulcus, it is important to seat it as far apically as safely possible before applying pressure. This gives you more leverage to push the entire root fragment instead of tipping it, which could cause the root tip to fracture (Fig 10-26).

You may find that reentering the sectioned area and cutting deeper between the root fragments may be required. Be aware that you are pressuring against the adjacent bone, so do this in a gentle manner, paying attention to the thickness and density of the adjacent bone. The mesial and distal bone is usually thicker than the buccal and lingual bone and therefore is less vulnerable to damage from instrument pressure.

If this does not mobilize the root fragments, it may be necessary to section them again, this time in the opposite (likely the buccolingual) direction. This is more applicable to larger roots, but smaller roots may require this step, at which time you are actually drilling out most of the root. Again, it is necessary to drill through the apex; feeling the bur drop into softer bone is an indication that you are past the apex. Enter the sectioned space with a thin elevator or an Orban knife and gently pressure the root fragments laterally. Then, pressure the sectioned fragments from the sulcus into the space created by sectioning the roots.

Once root segments are mobilized, lock onto an individual fragment with a hemostat or tweezers and use a gentle "wiggling" motion with constant pulling pressure to remove it from the socket (Fig 10-27). After one root section is removed, pressure the remaining root section with an Orban knife or thin elevator into the space created by removal of the first root section (Fig 10-28a). Then, remove the second root section (Fig 10-28b).

Once root removal is complete, proceed to socket debridement (see chapter 11).

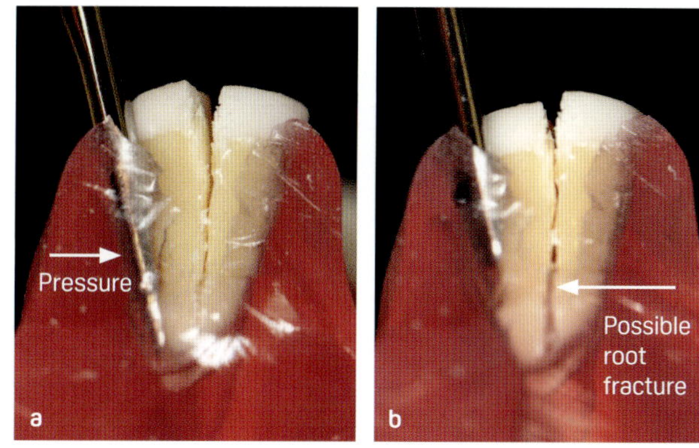

FIG 10-26 *(a)* Placement of thin Directa Luxator L2S elevator as far apically as possible at the buccal of the sectioned distal root to pressure rather than tilt it, reducing the risk of root fracture. *(b)* If the thin elevator is positioned only halfway down the root surface, there is a greater chance the root will fracture as it is pressured into the space created by sectioning the root. Pressure on the coronal half of the sectioned root stresses the mid-root area, leading to possible fracture, even if it is fully sectioned through the apex.

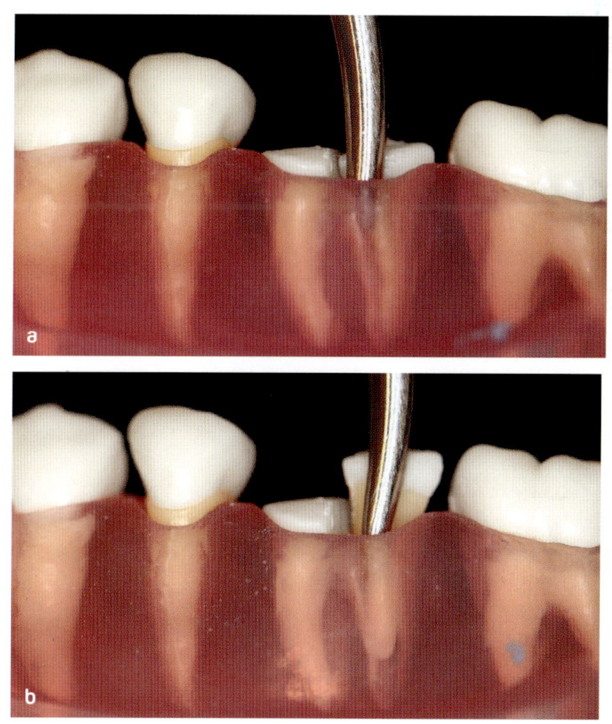

FIG 10-27 *(a and b)* Hemostat beaks are locked as far apically as possible on the buccal half of the distal root of the mandibular left first molar to remove it, using constant pulling pressure and a gentle back-and-forth motion.

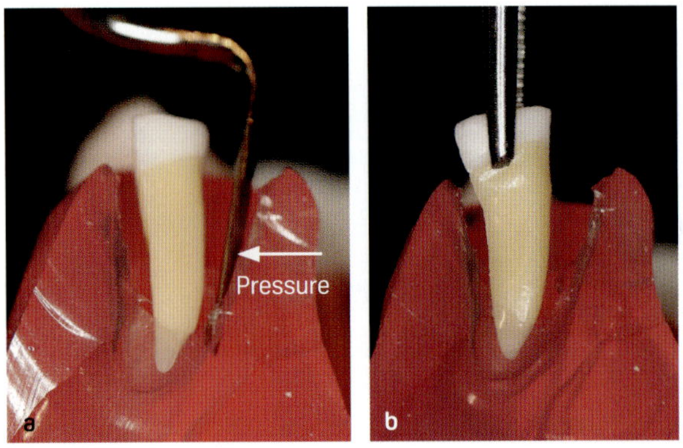

FIG 10-28 *(a)* Hu-Friedy Orban knife KO1/2IU placed at the apex of the remaining lingual half of the distal root, pressuring it into the space created by removal of the buccal half. *(b)* Once this remaining root half has been mobilized, it is removed with a hemostat or tweezers.

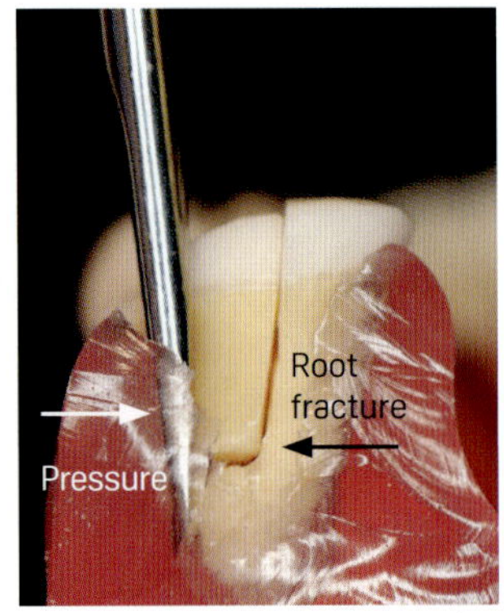

FIG 10-29 Thin Directa Luxator L2S elevator pressuring an incompletely sectioned distal root of the mandibular left first molar, resulting in horizontal fracture.

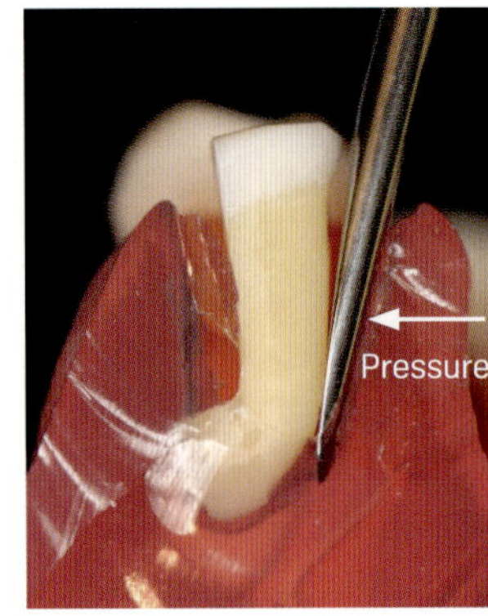

FIG 10-30 The thin Directa Luxator L2S elevator is used to pressure the remaining root, with the apex attached, into the space created by removing the root fragment (RSCET).

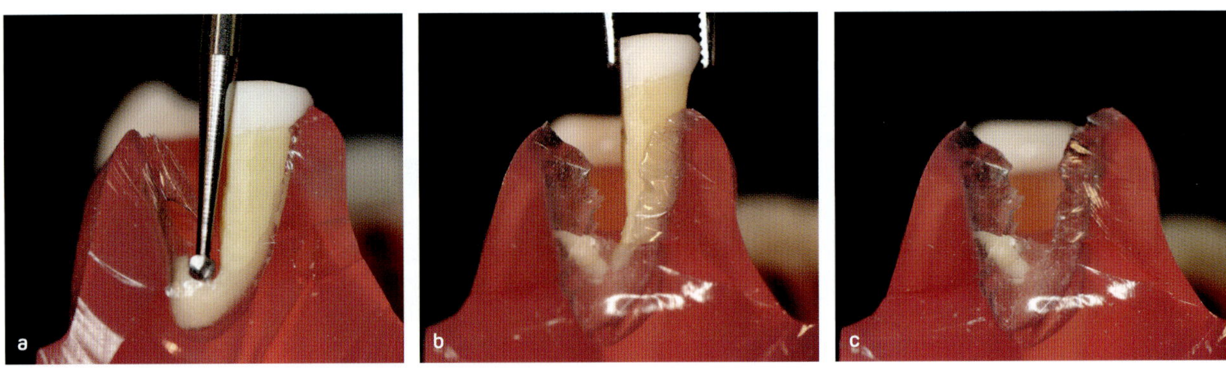

FIG 10-31 *(a)* If horizontal fracture occurs, remove the loose root fragment and use a straight handpiece bur #4 or #6 to completely section the root through the apex. Once through the apex, use an Orban knife to pressure the root half into the space created by removal of the root fragment. *(b)* Remove the long root fragment with tweezers. *(c)* Half apex remaining. This can be mobilized using a thin elevator and then removed with tweezers or by flushing with sterile saline.

Complications

If the root is not sectioned entirely through the apex or if the apex fractures, atraumatic removal is difficult. The following steps will help reduce the severity of such complications.

As mentioned earlier, if the root is not sectioned entirely through the apex, pressuring the root into the space may result in a horizontal fracture at the depth of the cut, leaving the apex attached to the remaining root (Fig 10-29). If horizontal fracture occurs, remove the loose root fragment. The choice is then to attempt to pressure the remaining root, with the apex attached, into the space created by removing the root fragment or to section through the apex.

If the remaining root is pressured into the space created by removing the root fragment (RSCET; Fig 10-30), the risk is another horizontal root fracture, leaving the entire apex. This approach is more successful in softer maxillary bone. Attempting this in the denser mandibular bone will result in fractures more frequently. The other option is to section through the apex (Fig 10-31).

A fractured apex is a complication we will all experience. Sectioning entirely through the apex is necessary to help prevent these complications.

Once root removal is complete, proceed to socket debridement (see chapter 11).

Socket Debridement

After the root(s) are removed, inspect for residual roots or root fragments, granulation tissue, and apical lesions. Rinse with chlorhexidine and saline, and use a long curet or periodontal probe to determine if all the bony walls are present and if and where granulation tissue remains. Look at a periapical radiograph of the area to determine if lateral bone loss or apical cysts are present. These are areas where granulation tissue will be present. Granulation tissue that fills areas of bone loss or lateral cysts should be removed because it may harbor bacteria or toxins. Once granulation tissue has been removed, bleeding will subside, and there will be less postoperative bleeding as well.

There are various methods of debriding the socket of granulation tissue. The most common method is the use of curets; however, this method has the following two negative features:

1. More time consuming
2. Patient hears a scraping noise

I believe the most efficient, least traumatic, and most thorough method is to first dissect granulation tissue away with a 15 blade (Fig 11-1). You can filet it away by scraping between the bony socket wall and the granulation tissue. At times it even can be removed in one piece. Next, use the straight handpiece round bur #10 with irrigation, and then use the smaller straight handpiece round bur #6 to debride the apex (Fig 11-2).

At this point, curets may be used to check for residual granulation tissue. Large and small curets can be used, as well as a 90-degree curet for defects lateral to the socket. Continue to irrigate with sterile saline

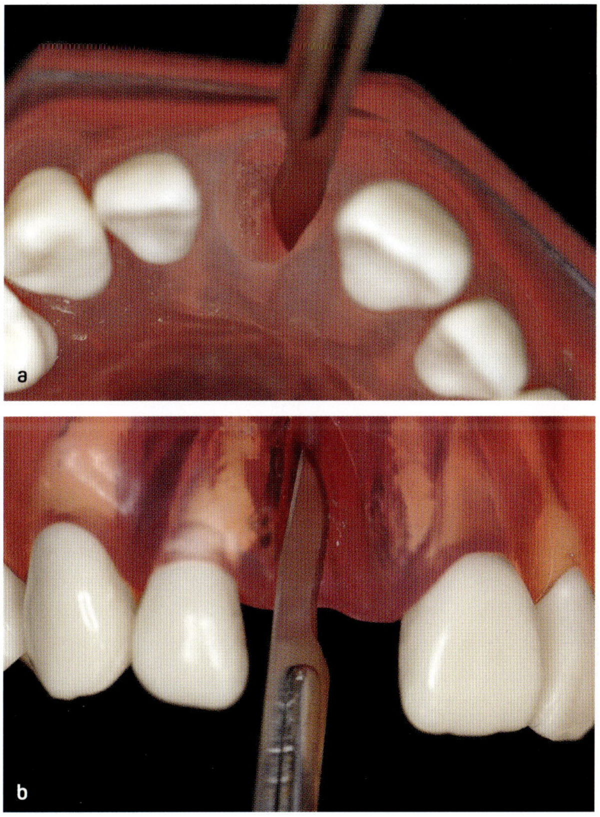

FIG 11-1 *(a and b)* A 15 blade used to dissect granulation tissue from the socket wall. This will cause less tugging, pulling, and trauma compared to a curet.

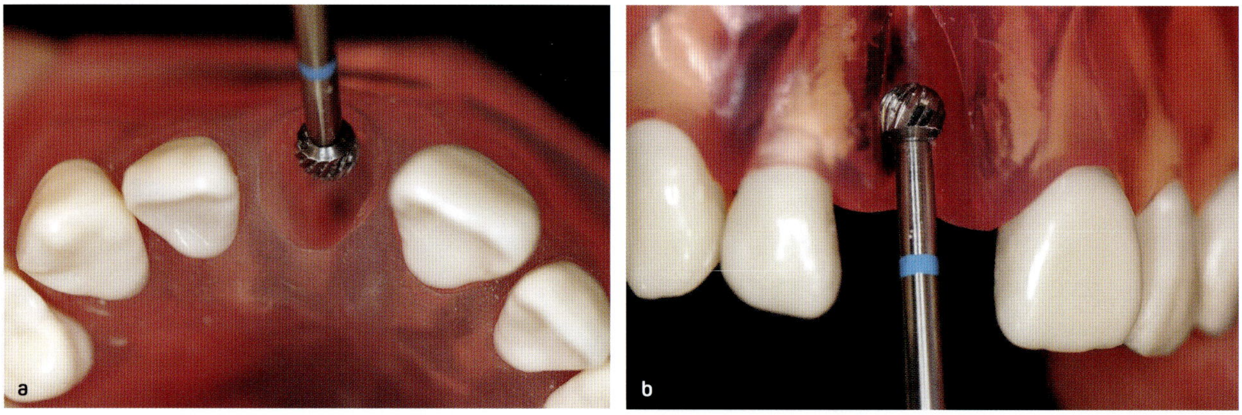

FIG 11-2 *(a)* A straight handpiece round bur #10 is used at low speed with an up-and-down motion to debride the maxillary right central incisor socket, removing periodontal ligament and granulation tissue. *(b)* Facial gingiva removed for better view.

and chlorhexidine and to inspect. I rinse the socket with chlorhexidine and then place 10% tetracycline gel for 1 minute. Then proceed to a socket preservation protocol if one is planned.

You may consider perforating the socket wall with a small round bur to increase blood supply to the site. This is similar to perforating the cortical bone when performing ridge augmentation. This is especially helpful if the socket wall is not porous or if bleeding is not evident.

To control bleeding, have the patient bite on a large 4×4 gauze, leaving one end hanging out of the mouth to prevent aspiration. A 2×2 gauze is too small and can be aspirated. A sedated patient will not be able to feel the gauze due to the anesthesia, and gauze is not visible on a radiograph, making it difficult to detect.

12

Using an Atraumatic Root Extraction Device

Commercial root extraction devices such as the Easy X-Trac System (A. Titan) and Benex Root Extraction System (Meisinger) can be used when there is an intact tapered root remaining with adequate width to allow a threaded rod to be inserted and have retention within the root.

This chapter presents the use of the Easy X-Trac System (Fig 12-1) to extract a maxillary left central incisor. To use the system, the crown first must be removed by horizontally sectioning the tooth 1 mm coronal to the gingival margin (Fig 12-2) as described in chapters 4 through 10. A hole is drilled into the root canal space (Fig 12-3), and a threaded rod is screwed into this hole (Fig 12-4). The protector plate is placed over the rod to serve as a base of leverage for the Easy X-Trac device (Fig 12-5). The Easy X-Trac device is placed on the protector plate and acts as a small jack to coronally pressure the threaded rod with the root attached, lifting the root out of the socket (Fig 12-6). Because the root is tapered (ie, wider at the coronal aspect), it can be removed from the socket with minimal damage to the bone of the socket wall (Figs 12-7 and 12-8).

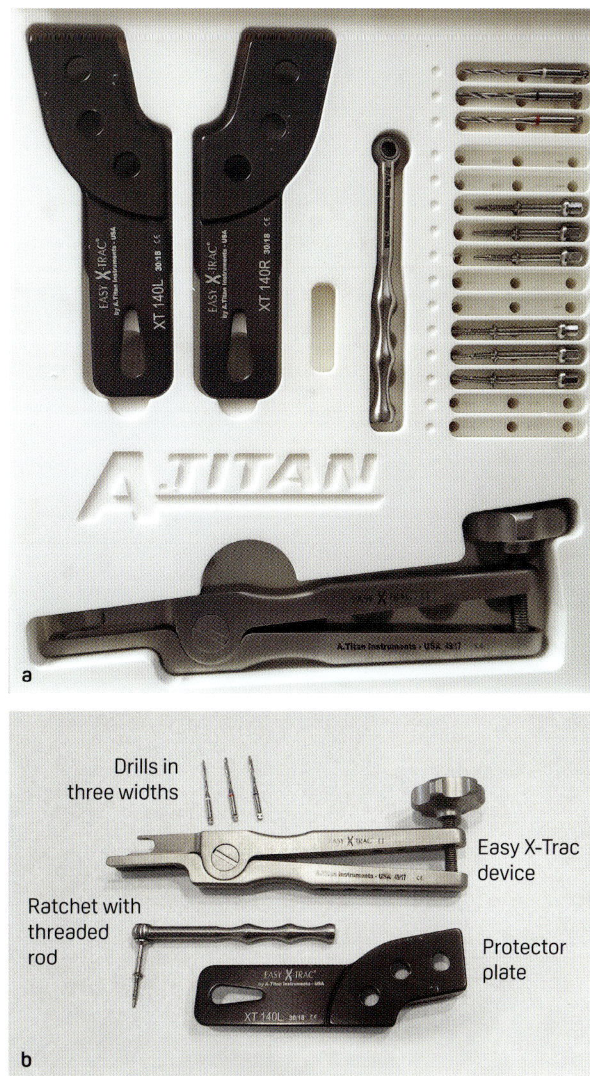

FIG 12-1 *(a and b)* Easy X Trac kit.

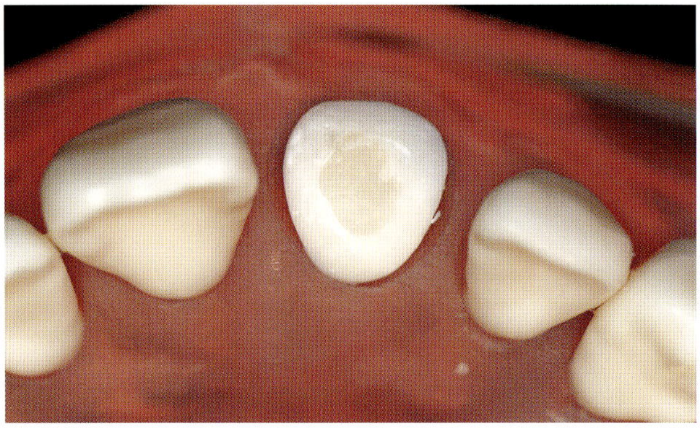

FIG 12-2 Maxillary left central incisor with crown removed by horizontal sectioning 1 mm coronal to the gingival margin.

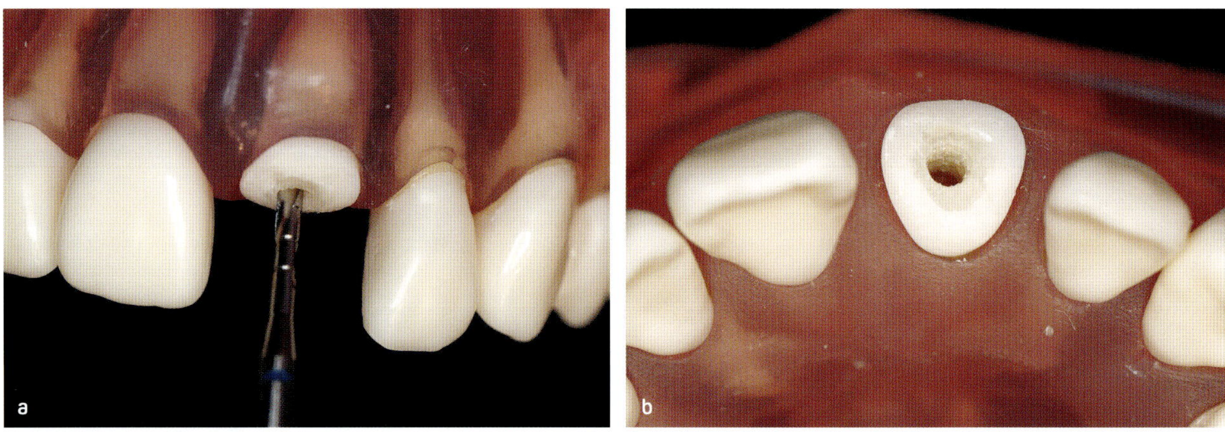

FIG 12-3 *(a and b)* Hole drilled into root canal space.

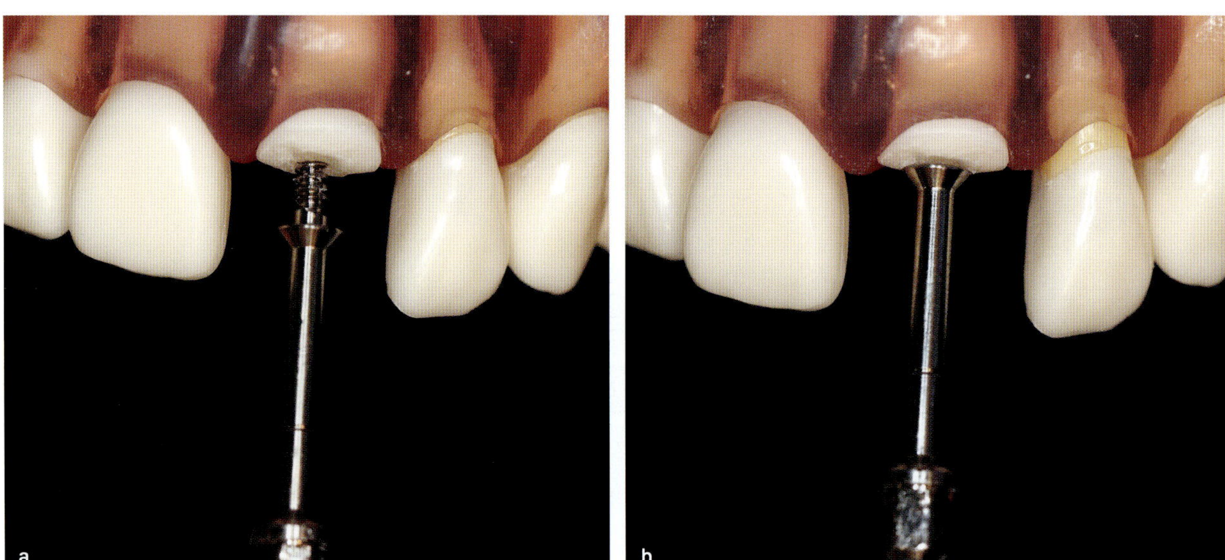

FIG 12-4 *(a and b)* Threaded rod screwed into the root canal space.

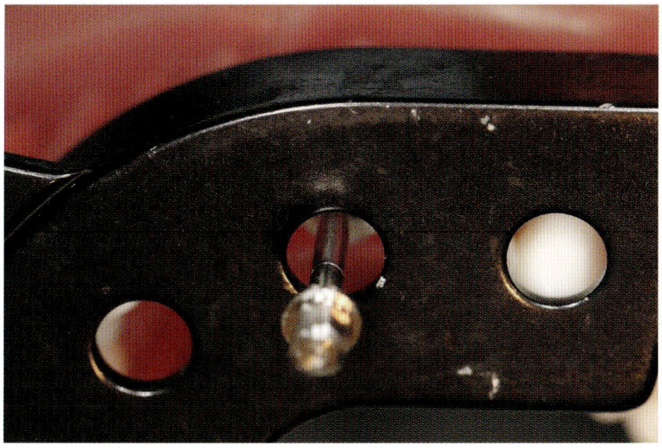

FIG 12-5 Protector plate placed over threaded rod to serve as a leverage base for the Easy X-Trac device.

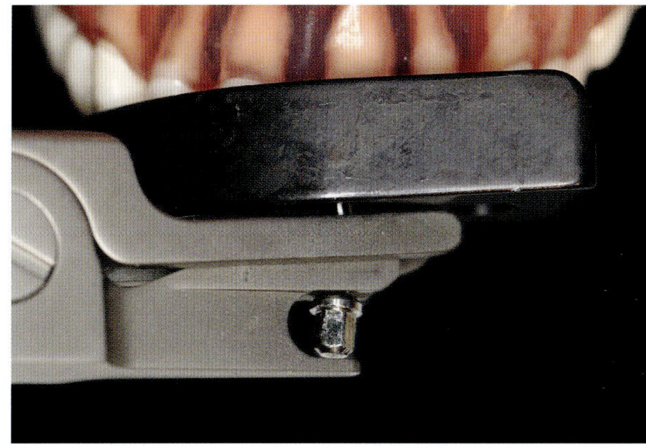

FIG 12-6 Easy X-Trac device used to remove the threaded rod with root attached. The device moves the threaded rod coronally, removing the root.

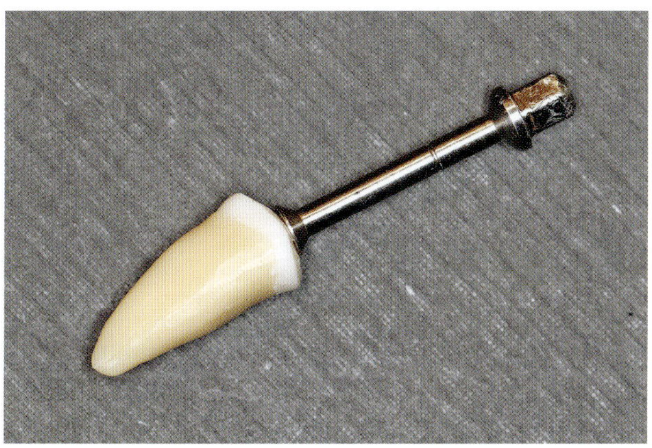

FIG 12-7 Root removed with threaded rod attached. This is an atraumatic extraction due to the tapered root.

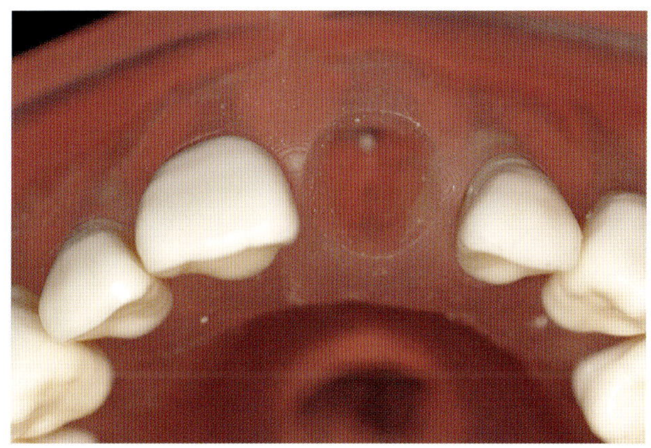

FIG 12-8 The socket is ready for socket preservation or implant placement.